# THE CLOUD AND THE LIGHT:

## MEMOIRS OF A JAPANESE CHRISTIAN SURGEON FROM NAGASAKI

by

MARTIN KAWANO, M.D.

Translated into English by Martin Kawano
from the Japanese Edition (1993)

# THE CLOUD AND THE LIGHT:

## MEMOIRS OF A JAPANESE CHRISTIAN SURGEON FROM NAGASAKI

by

MARTIN KAWANO, M.D.

Translated into English by Martin Kawano
from the Japanese Edition (1993)

Edited by Paul W. Miller, Ph.D.,
Professor Emeritus of English, Wittenberg University
in consultation with
William J. Chambliss, Ph.D.,
Professor Emeritus of History, University of Kentucky

Cross Cultural Publications, Inc.

CrossRoads Books

*The West and the Wider World Series, Volume XII*



Published by **CROSS CULTURAL PUBLICATIONS, INC.**
**Cross Roads Books**
Post Office Box 506
Notre Dame, Indiana, 46556, U.S.A.
Phone: (219) 273-6526, 1-800-561-6526
FAX: (219) 273-5973


ISBN: 0-940121-39-5
Library of Congress Catalog Card Number: 96-86628

# FOREWORD

As a doctoral candidate in English at the University of Michigan, I first met Dr. Martin Kawano at an Ann Arbor campus chapel in the fall of 1951, where he was studying on a GARIOA (precursor of the Fulbright) fellowship in the University's School of Public Health. Having been a Japanese medical student at the University of Nagasaki in 1945, where he miraculously survived the atomic blast of August 9 at only 700 meters from its epicenter, Martin came to the United States six years later as a lung surgeon fresh from Japan's post-war epidemic of tuberculosis. In the United States he wanted to learn advanced techniques of pulmonary surgery, preferably at the University of Michigan because of its fine reputation in the field. But as luck, or fate, or providence would have it, he had noted on his application form only that he wanted to study tuberculosis, not surgery, and so he was assigned by mistake to the School of Public Health. By June, 1952, he had obtained a Master's degree in public health administration, but not the clinical training he needed. Determined not to return to Japan without achieving his goal, Martin reluctantly decided to stay in the U.S. for one more year, far from his dear, loyal wife Miwa. Fortunately, he was able to obtain a residency at Glen Lake Sanatorium near Minneapolis, Minnesota, where he assisted with pneumonectomies on an almost daily basis, thereby obtaining the hands-on experience he needed. In the summer of 1953 he returned to Miwa and the little house she had built in his absence on land razed by the atomic blast. This is the house which Martin and Miwa still call home, and where Martin still carries on his private medical practice since his official retirement as a hospital administrator in 1986.

When I first met Martin in Ann Arbor, he was in his early thirties, but with his pale, almost ashen face, slim build and irrepressible chuckle he seemed younger than I; actually, he was several years older. Though I soon learned that he had survived the atomic blast, I did not know till years later that he had also survived three years of rigorous service in a Japanese cavalry regiment and two severe bouts of tuberculosis induced by inadequate diet and malnutrition during and soon after the war. Nor did I know till recently that he had been so poor in Ann Arbor, even with a fellowship, that for supper each night he was reduced to eating California rice mixed with green peas and ground meat colored with ketchup. We did not know of his hardship because he was too proud to tell us; he also must have been fearful of exploiting our friendship by accepting from us the food that we would have willingly shared with him on a more or less regular basis, in our tiny basement apartment. My wife Mary Jo and I still wince whenever we think of our insensitivity to his plight at that time.

Though he has remained thoroughly Japanese and proud of most aspects of Japanese culture, it would nevertheless be fair to say that like his native southern Japanese island of Kyushu, first opened to the West by the Jesuit missionary Francis Xavier in 1549, Martin has had a long love affair with the West. It began with his shocking conversion to Christianity at the age of thirteen as the seventh (and last) son of a poor but devout Buddhist baker, and continued in the course of eight post-World War II visits to the United States and/or Europe from 1951 to 1986, for a total of five years abroad. Martin spent most of his time abroad studying medicine in the United States. First, as noted above, he studied pulmonary disease and practiced lung surgery in the Midwest; then, after tuberculosis was brought under control in Japan by about 1958 with the aid of antibiotics, he developed his new specialty, brain surgery (or "nut cracking," as he sometimes jokingly called it) on the West Coast, first in Portland, Oregon and later in Loma Linda, California. (Back home he became so thoroughly identified with brain surgery that he was nicknamed Ben Casey of Nagasaki, after the popular TV neurosurgeon.) Even as he became an unofficial Japanese ambassador and interpreter of Japanese culture to Americans on these visits, I am confident that he also served as a sensitive, sympathetic interpreter of American life to his patients, acquaintances and society at large during his several decades of medical service in Japan. I also believe that Martin's memoirs will make a significant contribution to American understanding of Japanese culture, even as the second Japanese edition of his memoirs, published in 1993, will by now have replaced some of the Japanese myths and misinformation about the West with Martin's penetrating observations, based on his wide experience of life in different parts of the United States, Canada and Europe.

In the course of his visits abroad Martin became acquainted with several internationally famous surgeons and other notables, including the pioneer microsurgeon M.G. Yasargil and the brain surgeon Hugo Krayenbuhl, both of Zurich, the distinguished pianist Dr. Christiane Eckert Engel, who is Dr. Albert Schweitzer's granddaughter, now living in California, and the late Maria von Trapp of Stowe, Vermont, from whom the character of Maria in *The Sound of Music* was created. Martin's accounts of his encounters with famous people are invariably fresh, honest, and insightful. But although he has enjoyed the company of these people, he has never lost his sympathy for and understanding of the common, poor, uneducated people from which he sprang, or forgotten his Christian mission to minister to the unfortunate and downtrodden as well as the privileged and affluent in society.

In hindsight one cannot help wondering how much of Martin's westering impulse was activated by the Hiroshima and Nagasaki bombings, with their awesome implications for American power and technology, more overwhelming in their impact by far than the American warships steaming into Yedo (Tokyo) Bay in 1853-54 under Commodore Matthew Perry, which initiated Japan's eventual transformation from an inward looking, feudal society to an outward looking, modern, industrial society under the Meiji regime (1867-1912).

Along with his specialized professional skills in lung and brain surgery, Dr. Kawano has devoted himself to important national and international causes, including his pioneering work in the Japanese Anti-Smoking Campaign and in one of the first Japanese suicide prevention hotlines. In the context of the ongoing

American struggle to reduce smoking at home and abroad, and to clip the wings of the powerful tobacco companies and their minions in Congress, it is fascinating to observe, from Martin's vantage point, the Anti-Smoking struggle in Japan, where the courageous foes of tobacco have faced almost overwhelming odds, owing to the Japanese government's monopoly on tobacco and the concomitant billions of yen in taxes tobacco brings in every year. In Japan, even more obviously than in this country, the tobacco interests are exploiting customers and citizens for profit and tax money, even in the face of sickness, early death, and endless medical bills for the individuals addicted and afflicted, not to mention tobacco's many indirect costs to society.

Between 1951, when my wife and I first met Martin, and the fall of 1992, when we accepted a five week teaching assignment to a Japanese Lutheran college in Japan, our chief contact with Martin had been through annual Christmas letters. But in 1992 things changed. Throughout our teaching and touring visit to Kyushu Jo Gakuin College in Kumamoto prefecture on Martin's home island, we first enjoyed the boundless hospitality of Chancellor Andy Ellis, Professors Nobuyuki Takaki and Elizabeth Huddle, and Professor Eriko Toyama, a former student of mine at Wittenberg who had invited us to teach at her college. Then, towards the end of our visit, Martin arrived in his speedy little car to take us on a whirlwind tour of southern Kyushu, including the boiling hot springs of Mt. Unzen, over which early seventeenth century Japanese Christians had been suspended until they recanted or died as martyrs; the hill of Nishizaka in Nagasaki, where 26 Christians were crucified on February 5, 1597; and of course the Peace Park and Museum commemorating the death of some 74,000 in the bombing of Nagasaki on August 9, 1945. Two effects of this visit were to make me aware of the great natural beauty of Japan, and to heighten my appreciation of her rich, complex and often puzzling culture. A third effect has been to renew for me the biblical concept of Christianity as a religion of risk takers and potential martyrs in a country where less than one percent of society is openly Christian. Martin, throughout his long, eventful life, has been among those Japanese Christian risk takers. And he has found the risks taken to be more than justified by his firm belief in a Christ-centered Providence that has given his life a seamless web of purpose, however inscrutable, fearful or painful some of the individual threads of that life have been, and continue to be. Though neither a saint nor a martyr, he repeatedly exhibits in his memoirs the firm convictions and tough-mindedness of which, historically speaking, Christian martyrs have been made. For example, when asked by his new company commander in 1942, "As a citizen of the Japanese empire, which order do you follow first, the emperor's or Christ's?" he replied, "I don't think the Emperor would order me to do anything against the teaching of Christ." In this incident, as in many others, Martin is revealed to be wise as a serpent and innocent as a dove, but in addition, iron-willed. It is perhaps a tribute to the changing tenor of modern Japanese society, specifically to its growing tolerance of and respect for the individual conscience, that Martin has not had to pay the price of his convictions with blood, like those thousands of Japanese Christian martyrs in the first two centuries of the Tokugawa regime (1603-1867).

Paul W. Miller
September 8, 1996

# INTRODUCTION

Dr. Kawano's life is extraordinary—it is a life filled with miracles, tragedies and pioneer work, guided by the Christian ethics of Brotherhood (*Naechstenliebe*). Against the odds he miraculously survived the atomic bomb attack on Nagasaki, being very near its deadly center. His recollection of this horrifying event should be read by everybody—a most powerful warning to humanity never to let it happen again and to forever completely stop nuclear armament and nuclear testing.

Having known Dr. Kawano for 26 years, having worked for a short time as a medical intern under his direction and on several occasions having lived for a short period at his welcoming, heart-warming home in Nagasaki, I have gained a deeper insight into his personality and developed a profound admiration and respect for him and his work. Tirelessly, still today at an age past the average man's life expectancy, he is here for his patients, for his family, and for his friends; tirelessly, he is pursuing causes to better our lives, our environment. At his side is his guiding angel: his remarkable, devoted, sweet and loving wife Miwa, whom I deeply respect and love.

My grandfather, Albert Schweitzer, had a great influence on Dr. Kawano. His philosophy of "Reverence for Life" has found practical realization in Dr. Kawano's life and work. They are, in the true sense, spiritual brothers.

Christiane Engel, M.D., Ph.D.

# CONTENTS

## PART I



## PART II

## PART III



## PART IV

# PART I

# 1

# THE NINTH OF AUGUST

The day broke peacefully on the morning of the ninth of August. I woke up in the basement of the Nagasaki Medical School Hospital where I had stayed all night since the loud sound of the siren gave warning of an air raid before midnight. Our group of medical students were assigned to the Department of Ophthalmology to be ready for fire or casualties.

"Why don't you come to my house for breakfast?" Mochizuki asked me. He was my classmate and lived in a rented room near the hospital with his new wife whom he had married at Kagoshima shortly after the city was bombed by American bombers in April. He thought it was unsafe for Michiko to stay in Kagoshima, at the southern end of Kyushu Island, the most southerly of the Japanese home islands.

Michiko is a short woman with a soft smile. She welcomed me and prepared breakfast for us. She was not strong enough to be recruited to women's hard labor in wartime Japan. She was protected in the parsonage of Furumachi Church, where I was serving as a lay preacher, for a couple of months until she recovered her strength. We enjoyed our breakfast, chatted, joked with each other and ended in laughter, when another warning siren broke the morning air, calling us to our duty. Mochizuki and I went back to the hospital and ran into the basement as soon as the siren signaled that an air raid was imminent.

It was after nine o'clock when we learned that the danger was over. We went into the lecture room to listen to the lecture of our Dean on medical diagnosis. Professor Tsunowo, the Dean, looked exhausted. No wonder. He had just returned from Hiroshima on the sixth of August. When the train from Tokyo stopped suddenly before arriving at Hiroshima, he had walked through the debris of a burning city attacked by an unprecedentedly powerful bomb. Yesterday morning he had told us how terrible was the disaster caused by an unknown weapon, and warned us to be ready for the worst.

When his lecture ended, we moved to the Outpatient Clinic for our training on physical examination and diagnosis. Seven of us had been assigned to the Department of Surgery. None of us was absent, even though this month of August was a month of vacation in peacetime. We were requested to finish our medical course as soon as possible, sacrificing all our holidays and vacations. The army desperately needed more doctors.

No patient was in the waiting room this morning after repeated warning sirens. We sat in the history-taking room and had nothing to do but chat.

Shortly before eleven o'clock, I noticed Professor Kohei Koyano entering the examination room on the other side of the corridor. My classmate Sasaki and I followed him but others were still busy chatting.

Professor Koyano sat on his chair and started examining a patient who faced him on a chair. So no time was wasted. I picked up a blank medical record and stood behind the Professor to write down his words, because I saw no other doctor ready to help him take the patient's history. I listened to Professor Koyano's words with care. The time was two minutes past eleven.

At that moment, the room was filled with a dazzling, brilliant light, as if a thousand magnesium flashes were ignited all at once. Instantly I tried to lie down on the floor to avoid the following blast, which came so fast it threw my whole body into the air.

I landed on the floor, using my hands and knees to support my body. I could see nothing but dark smoke filling the entire building. I could not breathe. The smoke seemed to choke my throat and lungs to death. I thought I was going to die. I held my breath and closed my eyes. Many events from my past life flooded my thoughts. So this is the last of my days. If this is the Will of God, I must accept it, and leave the rest to Him. I prayed, "*Dear Father, I thank thee for all thy guidance of Grace in my short life. It is sad that I accomplished nothing. Forgive me, God, and accept my soul, I pray.*"

My heart was filled with peace. There was no sorrow, no regret, and no fear.

I could not keep my breath any longer. I gave up and inhaled. I thought I was dying. But I was not! I was still alive. I turned around and saw a dim light in the distance. I walked toward the light. There was a broken window with shattered glass. I climbed onto the bottom of the lower window frame and looked down.

What I saw far below the window was not the ground but a narrow concrete floor outside the basement. I felt dizzy. I would be crushed if I jumped down. But look! There was a stone staircase leading from the basement to the ground, and a small flat square in the middle of the steps. Taking a big risk, I jumped onto the white square spot. My landing was successful. I walked up the steps and reached the ground level outside the hospital.

It was a strange world that I saw there: evening twilight in the middle of this midsummer day, filled with a mist of yellow-brown dusk. It was like the Inferno which Dante Alighieri described in his *Divina Commedia*. Ghost after ghost walked through the dark, smoky haze in the depths of the earth without sunlight. Their faces were covered with black soot, leaving only white teeth and eyeballs for contrast. They walked like daydreamers with neither expression nor voice. They were apathetic yet seeking an escape. Their clothes were torn, exposing large areas of bruised skin. More and more passed by. And all of them were moving in silence towards the rear gate of the hospital leading to the hill behind, because beyond the front gate was the smoke and flame of the burning buildings around and below the Medical School Hospital. I realized that the distant sound of the tidal wave I heard was actually the desperate chorus of people in peril, thousands of voices shouting for rescue in vain.

I also heard a weak voice asking for help near my foot. I saw a nurse wearing a ripped, white uniform soaked with soot and dust. Her face was soiled and stained with blood. Her hair looked scorched. What a pitiful change for a white angel! I took her hand and carried her on my back and joined the line of ghosts. As we approached the rear gate, I saw a tall pillar of fire rising from the direction of the medical school campus, where our junior medical students had been studying this morning. I was shocked by the thought that those younger students were being burnt alive in those wooden buildings devoted to basic medical science.

Running away from the chorus of agonizing people in the pillar of fire, the current of silent ghosts went through the rear gate of the hospital and walked up the slope of the hill. Seeing the heavy burden on my back, another medical student offered me his help and took the wounded nurse on his back. I was relieved and followed them towards the hill, remembering the words of the Scripture:

*Then let them which be in Judea flee into the mountain:*

*Let him which is on the housetop not come down to take any thing out of his house: Neither let him which is in the field return to take his clothes.*

*And woe unto them that are with child, and to them that give suck in those days!*

*But pray ye that your flight be not in the winter, neither on the sabbath day. For then shall be great tribulation, such as was not since the beginning of the world to this time, no, nor ever shall be.*

*(Mt. 24:16-)*

These words of Christ in the first century came alive, as if he had predicted what happened today.

As I was meditating on this prophecy on the way, a small boy came into my sight. He was crying in front of a destroyed house. When I approached the place, I noticed a struggling foot sticking out from the edge of the fallen roof. I heard the voice of a woman shouting, “Help this child, please!"

I could not see the body which was under the debris of the house. It was impossible to rescue her without others' help. Yet the storm of flame was close behind me. There was no time to waste. I shouted in an agonizing voice “I'll save the boy. You don't have to worry," and took the hand of the boy, whose head was wounded and bleeding. I had to dress his wound quickly with my cotton legband. I tried to lead the crying boy with my hand, but more often I had to carry him on my back. We kept walking on the hillside. Our destination was the First Urakami Hospital where I used to attend the weekly round of the wards of tuberculosis patients. I wondered if Dr. Akizuki, the chief administrator, was safe. How would the patients and the nurses be? I had to go there as quickly as possible and help them.

Usually it took less than twenty minutes to reach the Hospital from the Medical School Hospital, but it took much longer that day, for there was not a single easy road. I had to find the way myself, and often had to detour because the road was blocked by debris from ruined houses. As the distance from the Medical School became longer, the air became a little cooler, and the smoke thinner, although the sky was still dark. It took time to walk with the wounded child, nearly two hours before I reached the Hill of Motohara and saw a lonely red brick building in smoke.

It was already three o'clock in the afternoon when I finally reached the hospital, carrying the sick child. The roof and floors of the hospital were burnt down. What I saw in the distance was the outer frame of the buildings, which had survived the fire. The fire was now burning the basement where medical supplies and food stocks were stored. Brother Iwanaga was busy pouring water onto the fire. He had to run for water again and again with his limping legs. Other people were holding their hands in despair. Immediately I ran toward Brother Iwanaga and offered my help, leaving the child to a Catholic sister. The two of us kept pouring water onto the fire until it finally died. We succeeded in salvaging food and medical supplies of vital importance.

Dr. Akizuki was safe and unhurt. But Miss Yoshioka, a female doctor, had her face cut by glass splinters. The head nurse, Sister Fukahori, was also wounded. Father Ishikawa had been hit on the head with a concrete block, but it was not a serious blow. No one was killed. Patients in the wards were evacuated quickly. The severely sick patients and those under the fallen debris were carried out to safety. Miss Murai, the nurse, was unhurt; acting quickly she used sound judgement in directing the male patients to help her. From a dark corner of the hospital, she saw me in the distance and smiled at me as if to congratulate me on my safe escape, even though I had my head bound to cover a bleeding wound. She looked like an angel in her white uniform, standing in the debris.

Dr. Akizuki was exhausted. He also had tuberculosis of the lung. Nevertheless, he had to work all day, running around to rescue patients under his care, often carrying the sick patients away from the building on fire. He kept working without lunch, treating their injuries and burns. He was sick himself. He felt desperate when he realized the loss of hospital wards and equipment and saw the flow of injured victims seeking help in the only hospital existing in the Urakami District, where he soon found that all private practitioners were dead or dying.

It was fortunate that the storage area in the basement survived the fire, because the hospital's stored food and some medical supplies were intact, thanks to Brother Iwanaga's initiative and endurance. It was encouraging that we had some things we needed for treatment, even though all the expensive x-ray machines were totally destroyed. At least we had a safeguard from the otherwise inevitable hunger and starvation, because one thousand raw rice bales were stored in the basement by order of the Prefectural Government.

Under the direction of Dr. Akizuki, a brick furnace was built, and the unpolished rice was cooked in a large iron pot. Rice balls and cups of soybean soup were handed to everyone in the open floor or the yard, and everyone was happy to have something to eat after a long day without food. Dr. Akizuki ordered that meals should be provided not only to patients, nurses, brothers, sisters and seminary students, but also to every sick person, even to uninjured neighbors who took refuge in the hospital premises. It was not until a few days later that rice balls prepared by the city rescue teams reached this Urakami district of total destruction.

Complete darkness took over the dim light of the day, but the fire was still burning and smouldering in the Urakami District. A big flower of sparks blossomed in the dark sky and then sank into the silhouette of the huge Urakami Cathedral, the largest in Asia, as its buildings collapsed one after another. There were many corpses still burning. In the stream near the cathedral, there were the floating bodies of those who drowned when they jumped in fleeing from the unbearable heat and burns. Nevertheless, the night was calm and quiet, without any sound of human voices. All lying on the grass around me were in deep sleep. They were exhausted. No strength was left to think about tomorrow. Yet Dr. Akizuki was called often to examine the severely wounded patients. Intermittently came a weak, tearful voice from the small boy I had carried. "The wound must hurt him, and he misses his mother," I thought.

It had been a long day. It was hard to believe that I was here alive.

It could be nothing but Providence. The words of Psalm 91 came to my mind:

*Thou shalt not be afraid for the terror by night; nor for the arrow that flieth by day;*

*Nor for the pestilence that walketh in darkness; nor for the destruction that wasteth at noonday.*

*A thousand shall fall at thy side, and ten thousand at thy right hand; but it shall not come nigh to thee.*

Nagasaki was not included in the original plan as a target of the atomic bomb. Four cities were selected at first; Kyoto, Hiroshima, Yokohama and Kokura. Later, Kyoto was removed from the list and Niigata was added. It was on the night of the 24th of July, one week after the success of the experiment in Los Alamos, that Nagasaki was finally added to the list.

A heavy bomber,"Bock's Car," loaded with a plutonium bomb, flew up in the sky from Tinian, one of the Mariana Islands, early in the morning on the ninth of August. Their first target was Kokura in northern Kyushu and the second was Nagasaki, in western Kyushu. The sky over the city of Kokura was covered with cloud. Major Chuck Sweeney gave up the attack upon Kokura and turned the plane's nose to Nagasaki. As soon as Captain Kermit Beahan, the bombardier, recognized the Mitsubishi Arms Factory along the Urakami River through a gap in the clouds, he dropped the atomic bomb. It was two minutes after eleven.

The bomber climbed up at full speed. After forty seconds, the bomb exploded in the air, 500 meters above the Urakami River, at the midpoint between Nagasaki Medical School and Matsuyama Primary School, each situated 500 meters from the epicenter. Explosion of the "Fat Man," a plutonium bomb equivalent to 21 kilotons of TNT, a bomb much more powerful than the uranium bomb dropped on Hiroshima, immediately created an ultraheat of several million degrees and a mammoth fire ball of 300,000°C. Heat and radiation including infra-red rays burned all human beings and animals to cinders within a radius of one kilometer from the center, causing fire in a wide area. Even the exposure of the skin to the heat outside of a three kilometer radius left burns on the skin.

Ultra-pressure of hundreds of thousands pounds of barometric air pressure caused a bomb blast of 440 meters per second, smashed all buildings in the 500 meter radius, and destroyed wooden buildings within one and a half kilometers of ground zero, as the epicenter of the blast was called. Many people were crushed by the blast and many others were burnt to death under the debris of buildings. Survivors of the blast and fire thanked their good luck only temporarily. Another menace followed them—the unexpected killer, radiation!

Released gamma-rays in the center of the explosion were 25,100 rads.They were 7,090 rads in the medical school campus, 500 meters from the center, and 3,110 rads in the Medical School Hospital, 700 meters from the epicenter, and 888 rads at a distance of one kilometer. There was no chance of survival, once one was exposed to these fatal doses. I was not killed because the outpatient clinic was inside the reinforced concrete building, and five minutes before the explosion I had moved to the examination room whose window was facing toward the harbor instead of toward the center of explosion. My classmate Michio Katayama, who remained in the other room, was injured severely and jumped out of the window. His dead body was found later outside of the basement.

It was reported that 73,884 citizens died in Nagasaki. No one survived within the 500 meter radius from the hypocenter. Only five percent of the people between the 500 and 1,000 meter radii survived. Forty out of 70 undergraduates died. One third of my classmates, the third year medical students, died. My old pal Muneo Araki was killed with all his second year classmates and Professor Umeda, who was giving a lecture on pathology at 11:02. None of the first year students who attended the class had any chance of survival. Many professors were also victims of the Nagasaki bomb. Dean Tsunowo, who informed us of the disaster in Hiroshima, died two weeks later as the result of heavy radiation. The total number of casualties in the Nagasaki Medical School and Hospital was 892, including 17 professors, 10 associate professors, 15 lecturers, 535 medical students, 109 nurses and 206 other employees. Many of them were victims of radiation.

# 2

# MISERICORDIA

Near the Government Office of Nagasaki Prefecture, there stands a stone sign with an inscription: "Once here was the Misericordia." One can find this sign if one walks only one minute to the east from the Grand Hotel. It was there that the volunteer group named "Misericordia" opened the "Hospitalium" for the sick and the "Jihiya" or Charity House, for the old and the orphans in 1570, one year before the Port of Nagasaki was opened. It was the best "Misericordia" institute in Japan, although a similar institution had been in Yamaguchi, the western end of Honshu Island, since 1554. Also Brother Armeida had started a hospital and an orphanage in Oita, Kyushu, in 1556 with the help of twelve young Japanese male nurses.

According to the 1590 Annual Report of Father Frois, 120 members headed by a Japanese named Justino, collected donations and operated homes for the old, for the widows and for the lepers. Justa, the wife of Justino, and twelve other women took care of the deserted patients as pioneer nurses in Japan. The number of Hospitali increased to seven at its peak. Besides the Hospitalium and Jihiya, there was "Zeniya," a pawn shop for the poor, to save poor people from the merciless money lenders.

Lord Omura Sumitada was baptized in 1562 and helped missionaries in their mission work, defying the opposition of his subordinates. In ten years, nearly all 60,000 residents in his territory became Christians. They comprised 40 percent of all the Christians in Japan at that time. When Sumitada donated the city of Nagasaki to the Society of Jesus in 1578, all the citizens were Christians. The executive members of the "Misericordia" included the names of famous leaders of the city, Thomas Goto and Joan Machida.

Misericordia means "mercy" in Latin, the warm heart of mankind. It is the heart (*cordia*) which aches with sympathy and aspires to help the miserable (*miser*). "Misericordia" was first organized in Florence, Italy, in 1240. It was later organized on the Iberian Peninsula in 1498, and Santa Casa de Misericordia in Lisbon has been its headquarters until today. "Misericordia" spread to Goa and Macao as Portugal expanded her dominance to the Far East. It was organized in Japan, not only in Nagasaki, Yamaguchi and Oita, but also in Kyoto, Sakai, Arima, Ikitsuki and Kabashima. This organization fought against misery and cruelty in the period of constant wars in Japan in the 16th century,

The commandments of the "Misericordia" were "Fourteen Orders of Grace." One can discover these orders in the old Oratio memorized by "hidden Christians," or underground Catholics in Ikitsuki Island, northwest of Nagasaki, generation after generation surviving four centuries of persecution.

The "Fourteen Orders of Grace" consisted of two parts, "Seven Manners" and "Seven Spirits". The "Seven Manners" order:

1. Give food to the hungry.
2. Give water to the thirsty.
3. Clothe the naked.
4. Visit the sick.
5. Give shelter to travellers.
6. Receive the released prisoners.
7. Bury the dead.

These "Manners" call for nothing but the practice of the words of Christ in St. Matthew (Chapter 25:35-). Four hundred years ago in Nagasaki Japanese Christians were practising what Mother Teresa has been doing with the members of the Missionaries of the Love of God in Calcutta.

However, this activity had to be discontinued. Suddenly in 1587, on the 24th of July, Toyotomi Hideyoshi, who had earlier been in favor of Christianity, gave a decree prohibiting Christianity. Overnight, Christianity became a forbidden religion and all Catholic missionaries were ordered to leave Japan. The famous Christian Lord, Takayama Ukon, was stripped of his land when he refused to convert to Buddhism. Thereafter, the decree was not reinforced by Hideyoshi. He even enjoyed the occidental music played by the Catholic boys who came back to Japan from the nine-year-long journey to Europe to visit the Pope in Rome. A new wave of persecution was ignited by a Spanish ship, "San Felipe," which drifted ashore on the Southern beach of the Shikoku Island. Hideyoshi ordered the arrest of missionaries and Japanese Christians after hearing the boast of a sailor that the ultimate goal of Catholic Missions was the subjugation and occupation of nations, as demonstrated in the Philippine Islands. Twenty-four Christians including Franciscan Father Pedro Baptista were arrested by the Kyoto Marshal Ishida Mitsunari on December 8, 1596. There were boys among them: 12-year-old Rudobico, 13-year-old Antonio and 14-year-old Thomas. All twenty-four Christians had their ears cut off and were chased through the streets of Kyoto. They were then forced to walk a long way to Nagasaki on foot in the cold winter. On the way, two more Catholics volunteered to join them. In all, twenty-six Christians were finally crucified at Nishizaka, a hill looking over the harbor of Nagasaki, on the 5th of February, 1597.

Two hospitals in Kyoto were closed, and the "Misericordia" in Kyoto disappeared. However, the "Misericordia" in Nagasaki continued their work much longer. In 1614 the Shogun ordered another strict ban on Christianity. All missionaries were expelled from Japan, and all churches were destroyed, but the Jihiya and the Hospitalium in Nagasaki were spared. It was not until 1620 that they were destroyed at last, and the patients and the homeless were moved to private homes.

Merciless persecution began in 1625 uder the reign of Governor Mizuno and the Police Commander Suetsugu Heizo in Nagasaki. Those who refused to reconvert to Buddhism were driven out of the city with only one bag of rice. If they refused to leave the city, they had to starve to death in their homes, locked by the police. If they ran to the mountains, they would die of starvation in the end. Even in these inhuman circumstances, members of the "Misericordia" did not give up their activity until Migeru Kusuriya, their leader, was burned to death as a martyr on the 28th of July, 1633, 63 years after the onset of "Misericordia."

Miraculously, "Misericordia" revived in Urakami 312 years later, in the summer of 1945. Faced with the greatest misery in human history, with their *cordia* vibrating with sympathy, all Urakami Catholic survivors devoted their bodies and souls to help every miserable victim of the atomic bomb. The First Urakami

Hospital, which is now called St. Francisco Hospital, was the center of this new "Misericordia." I happened to be there as a witness, and helped their work for a month.

The only physician who survived in the Urakami district, where more than 12,000 Catholics lived, was Dr. Akizuki. Other doctors were killed or wounded by the bomb in their clinics. The only hospital remaining in this district was the First Urakami Hospital, standing with its burnt frames and walls. The Medical School Hospital was destroyed and burnt down, leaving wounded doctors and medical students who needed help for themselves. It took time to set up a new Emergency Medical Center in a primary school building in the center of the city, far from Urakami. Consequently all injured survivors in the Urakami district had to wait indefinitely for rescue. Only those who were able to walk left the inferno on foot and walked out seeking for help and treatment. There were left in the vast ruin many wounded people and the corpses.

Many were lying on the ground wounded and some were inside the ruined houses, waiting for help. Some others were still hiding and groaning in the air raid shelters. With the help of a seminary student and a few uninjured inpatients of the hospital I carried the wounded ones to the hospital. Dr. Akizuki went out whenever he was asked to examine patients outside the hospital. He was nearly exhausted, and I had to substitute for him sometimes.

The First Urakami Hospital standing alone on a hill became a refuge and an encouraging hope for those who were seeking help. Those with minor wounds walked up by themselves. Those with severe injuries were carried by families and neighbors. Rescue teams sent from the army and the city brought the wounded patients to the hospital and left them in a hurry. More than three hundred patients were put together on the ash floor without a roof. Many others had to stay in the back yard and on the road.

There was no time to be wasted on the dying patients. We treated those who needed immediate help first. Bleeding had to be stopped quickly. Many wounds were caused by pieces of broken glass or concrete. We had to remove them one after another. I cannot forget the sight of the uncountable number of glass pieces stuck in the naked back of a nurse when she removed her burnt, torn clothes. It took a very long time for me to remove all the bloody pieces from her body.

I was surrounded often by the low voices of prayer here and there:

*Hail Mary, full of grace. The Lord is with thee. Blessed art thou among women, and blessed is the fruit of thy womb, Jesus. Holy Mary, Mother of God, pray for us sinners, now and at the hour of our death. Amen.*

*Jesus, Maria, Joseph, I give you my heart and soul. Jesus, Maria, Joseph, assist me in my last agony. Jesus, Maria, Joseph, may I breathe my soul in peace with you. Amen.*

Other voices joined them saying "*Amen.*" Prayers never stopped at night. They were repeated, and ended with the final prayer: *"May the souls of the dead rest in the Grace of our Heavenly Father."* The sound of sobbing followed.

Dr. Akizuki and I felt helpless and sad. The only comfort was the fact that those unfortunate victims were surrounded by compassionate hearts and were taken to Heaven assisted by many prayers.

After crying and missing his mother for two full days, the boy I had rescued became silent and died before the sun rose on the third day. I could not carry out my promise to his mother, but his death was better for him than his continuing, unrelieved suffering. Sister Fukahori and Miss Murai, who tried to console him all the time, had tears in their eyes. Brother Iwanaga and seminary student Noguchi collected lumber and cremated this poor child in the back yard of the hospital, where more and more dead bodies were brought in and cremated on the open ground, day after day.

Many patients had burns to the skin, causing them to cry from pain. Severe, extensive burns could kill them. But I tried to dress the burns of each one. It made my back painful to sit near the patients lying on the floor, treating their wounds for many hours a day in a bending posture. There were so many patients and I had to treat them with the help of Miss Murai, who never complained about her pain or fatigue but kept her warm smile all the time.

Patients were many but the medicine and dressing materials were few. We suffered from a shortage of medical supplies. There was no way to get them unless I went out to get them myself. The

Prefectural Government building was burnt down, but there must be set up a rescue center in the intact area of the city where I could get medical supplies. I decided to try. I left the hospital and walked toward the center of the city, passing by the ruined Urakami Cathedral.

The heat of the summer sun was unbearable even under the summer hat that I borrowed. More unbearable was the odor of corpses lying on the ground. When I reached a small river near the Urakami Cathedral, I saw several bodies floating on the water. The sight of a dead mother and a baby connected by the umbilical chord shocked me. Miscarriage must have occurred when the mother jumped into the water to escape fire and heat. I hurried and left the stream behind me, but I could not help seeing many burnt bodies scattered around.

I noticed living people walking among the corpses. They carried sacks on their backs and had water bottles hanging from their shoulders. They were searching for their dear ones or relatives. They turned the face of every apparently dead body upwards to see if it was the one they were looking for. But not all the bodies were dead. When raised for the check, one whispered, "Water. Please, water!" Another asked, "Do you have anything to eat?" when he heard steps. But the pedestrians walked away with obvious disappointment as soon as they saw that the speakers were strangers.

There must have been rice balls in the searchers' sacks. Their bottles must have been filled with water. But their food was not for strangers. Their water was not for the unknown. Their food and drink had to be saved for the ones they were desperately seeking. No food, no water would be given to any stranger before they found their dear ones. Their cold eyes showed their determination. Their love was only for their family or relatives. It was denied to strangers even if they were dying with thirst and hunger. It was the kind of love colder than the love of a demon. The scene made me sick, if not angry. My heart ached to realize this ugly aspect of human affection. I approached the one who asked for water, and helped him drink water out of my bottle. He drank it, and drank it with a joyful noise, and whispered in a husky voice, "This is the first sip of water I have had since that day."

Other bodies, not yet dead, heard our conversation, and looked at me with desperate eyes. I gave water to the one next to me. He did not thank me in words, but his eyes told me, "Thank you so much." He nodded and closed his eyes. I tried to give water to as many of the thirsty as possible, until my bottle became empty. I happened to find a water tap of dripping water. I filled the bottle with water and walked to the bodies on the ground to give them water if they were still alive. I wanted to give water to all who were suffering of thirst, but there were too many. I could not stay there all day, because I had an errand to secure medical supplies. I had to leave the place feeling sorry for others to whom I could not give water. Nevertheless, I thanked God for the opportunity of giving the last water to those who had to die in despair amid the ruins with no one around. The Lord promised: *"And whoever gives one of these little ones but a cup of cold water to drink... I assure you he will not lose his reward" (Matthew 10:24).* I learned that sometimes it is not easy to give a cup of water.

The meager medical supplies I had collected from the Emergency Center in the city did not last long. The need was much greater. That is why I jumped with joy when I heard we might obtain some supplies at the army hospital in Takematsu, Omura, 30 kilometers north of Urakami, where Captain Fukahori, a relative of Sister Fukahori, worked as a pharmacist. On the morning of August 15, I walked a long way to Michinoo Station, the next train station from Urakami, to catch an overcrowded train. The train stopped on its way when an American aircraft was spotted in the air, but there came neither shooting nor bombing. The train moved slowly again, and finally reached Takematsu Station shortly before noon.

In the army hospital, soldiers were ordered to line up in front of a radio, which reported that an important announcement was to be made by the Emperor. I joined them to listen to the broadcast. It started, but with too much noise. One could hardly understand what was said, but it was the voice of our Emperor. His sad tone and tension reflected the painful content of his message. It must be the announcement of surrender, the end of the war. No longer did we need to fear the aircraft in the air. I went back to Nagasaki on the train with a feeling of relief and safety.

It was in the evening at dusk when I arrived back at the First Urakami Hospital. I reported to Dr. Akizuki,"It's an unconditional surrender. I heard the announcement of the Emperor."

"Well, the end has come at last." He said no more, and continued his work in silence. I left the hospital to relay this news to Professor Koyano, acting Dean of our Medical School. I found him in the basement of the ruined Medical School Hospital, treating the injured medical students lying on the concrete floor. After listening to my report, he dropped his eyes and said nothing.

# 3

# ATOMIC DISEASES

"If they had accepted one week earlier the conditions of the Potsdam Declaration calling for Japan's unconditional surrender, this tragedy could have been avoided!" must have been the thought of Professor Koyano at that moment. He felt anger toward the irresponsible Japanese Army, which failed to end the war earlier. He also felt disappointment with the unwise government which had trusted Soviet Russia to act for peace negotiation with the allied forces. These thoughts must have made his heart sick and painful.

He was in the same room as I when we were attacked by the bomb. He was able to escape from the building, although his forehead and elbow were injured. Immediately he started treatment of the wounded in the underground shelter. On the following day he took command of the medical school as the acting Dean at the request of the wounded Dean, Professor Tsunowo. He built his headquarters in a shelter behind the hospital kitchen and treated wounded doctors and students who were brought in. He tried to rescue as many as possible from the burnt and ruined buildings. He also tried to grasp the whole situation and tried to make contact with the city authorities and rescue teams. He was too busy to see his home and his wife, who had little chance of survival.

It was only one month since he had moved to a new house in Shiroyama, near the Urakami River, from his old home, which was quite far from the Urakami district. His new home was only 700 meters from the hypocenter and was destroyed completely, while his old house in Rokasu-machi was intact. My father's house in nearby Shindaiku-machi and the Furumachi Church where I lived and worked since January were also intact.

Mrs. Koyano was not killed at once. She was rescued from her badly damaged house and carried to a downtown hospital. This news was a relief to Professor Koyano, but he worried about his wife's reportedly severe injury and fatigue. As the acting Dean, however, he could not leave the medical school to visit his wife. Anger toward the irresponsible war leaders and anxiety about his wife must have coexisted in his mind when he heard the news of the cease-fire.

At the end of the first week, Dr. Akizuki and I noticed unusual symptoms: hematuria and hemorrhagic stool. First, the patients found blood in their urine, then bloody diarrhea. The red color deepened, and frequency of elimination increased, and then they became increasingly emaciated and died. We suspected dysentery and felt helpless because we had no remedy for dysentery. A series of other alarming signs followed. Bleeding from the gums, loss of hair, and red spots all over the skin developed after the recovery from the direct damage of the bomb. If the red spots became purple, if bloody urination and bloody diarrhea persisted, transfusion of blood was useless. As soon as the needle of the injector was pulled out of the vein, the blood leaked from the hole in the vein. These symptoms were the result of severe radiation and the collapse of the vascular system. Red and white blood cells and platelets were lost in the body. We thought we had survived in the dangerous zone of radiation, but we might develop radiation disease as they did. Dr. Akizuki was exposed at a distance of 1,500 meters and I was at 700 meters from the hypocenter. We were terrified.

Around this time Dr. Nagai, our Associate Professor of Radiology, was treating the sick people at his headquarters of the Mitsuyama Rescue Center in Kobago village, one kilometer north of Urakami. He kept detailed medical records of the 125 patients he treated in 58 days from August 14 to October 8. This document was discovered 25 years later and was published in 1970 by Asahi News Press with the title of "A Report of the Atomic Bomb Diseases."

"In the second week, a few cases of sudden bleeding to death were found among those cases of severe post-radiation anemia. In the fourth to the eighth week, petechiae, small purplish red spots, were found in many of those who were exposed to the atomic bomb radiation at a distance between 500 meters and 1000 meters from the hypocenter. Petechiae were found also in those who were buried in the destroyed houses for hours and those who stayed in the shelters or temporary barracks for a few days. They looked healthy at first and worked to remove the debris. But gradually they became anemic, complained of general malaise, and suddenly developed high fever, painful rice-sized whitish spots and inflammation in the mouth. The gums bled easily and became necrotic and dark purple in color. Oral intake became difficult or impossible due to the severe pain inside the mouth. The greenish pale skin disclosed many spots of red bean color, starting from the trunk and upper arm, then spreading to the whole body, especially over the thighs. Their size varied from a pin size to the size of rice or bean. Some of them grew to the size of the small finger."

Dr. Nagai was exposed in his room in the Radiology Department on the second floor of the medical school hospital at a distance of 700 meters. He was hit by the blast and was injured. Compressing the bleeding wound of his scalp, he rescued his staff buried under the debris. He formed a rescue team of his own and saved many lives, working endlessly without taking rest for three days. In the evening of August 11, he went home for the first time. All he found in his house was a black scorched mass. When he picked up the mass, scorched bones collapsed and a rosary fell onto the ashes. He picked up the skull and pelvis of his wife, and put them in a bucket. When he sat down and embraced the bucket, he fell into coma.

He had had leukemia already. When he joined the Department of Radiology in 1932, the Roentgen machine was still using a naked tube without protective devices. After the onset of the Sino-Japanese War, his colleagues were drafted one after another, and Dr. Nagai was left alone to do all radiological examinations. Single-handed, he sometimes examined as many as several hundred men in a single day. Near the end of the war, film was not available any more. He had to copy the fluoroscopic findings on papers during examination. It was just a matter of time before a radiation disturbance due to overexposure to many kinds of harmful rays developed. Dr. Nagai himself suspected leukemia and confirmed enlargement of his liver on the radiogram in June, 1945. His white bloodcell count was 105,000, fifteen times the normal count. Exposure to the atomic bomb radiation at a short distance aggravated his leukemia, as one can guess, and his unexpected hard work in the three following days exhausted him. He thought he would die soon.

The next morning, however, he woke up. He was not dead. He picked up the bucket containing the bones of his wife and walked to the north until he reached Fujinowo village, where his two children, a 12-year-old boy and a 6-year-old girl, were waiting for the return of their parents in their grandparents' house. On the day after his arrival at Fujinowo, he started his long rescue work with his rescue team.

Miraculously he survived six more years. He stayed in his small hut, which he built in the ruined ground of his old house, and named "Nyokodo" after the commandment of Christ, "*Thou shalt love thy neighbour as thyself.*" "Nyoko" means "as thyself." The hut was only 36 square meters in size. In this small hut he wrote, and later dictated, twelve books. He taught the value of peace to the Japanese readers through his books, *The Bells of Nagasaki*, *The Chain of the Rosary* and others. He was called"A Saint in Urakami." He met many visitors, including the Emperor, in his humble hut where he stayed until his death on May 1, 1951.

Our Dean, Professor Susumu Tunowo, was examining a patient in the outpatient clinic when the atomic bomb exploded. His back was wounded by many splinters of glass, and his leg was injured. On the back of a young colleague he escaped to the hill behind the hospital. Professor Shirabe, a surgeon, treated his wounds. After staying overnight on the hill, he returned to the shelter in the hospital and stayed there until he was moved on a truck to a suburban shrine with other wounded colleagues during the evening of August 12. Professor Yamane was with him but died on the 15th after a series of tetanus convulsions. Professor Tsunowo watched him die in the same room. He looked better, but diarrhea started and his temperature went up. Still he was optimistic, telling his wife, "My dear, we shall go back to our hometown and start a private clinic as soon as I regain my strength."

On the nineteenth, he noticed petechiae and stomatitis. Gradually he lost consciousness, and on the twenty-second, death came to this great scholar of medicine. It was the result of "the atomic disease" caused by radiation from the atomic bomb.

Professor Shirabe was discouraged by the death of the Dean he had treated from the beginning. He had to close the rescue center at Iwaya after the Dean's death, because patients and nurses left Nagasaki when they heard that American forces were coming to occupy the city. For the first time after the bombing, Professor Shirabe found time to go back to the medical school to search for his second son, a first-year student of the school of medicine. Nothing but the stone foundation was left in the ruins of the school. In the sky, hundreds of crows were flying, madly looking for carrion from the dead human bodies. A few groups of scorched human bones had been accumulated, but there was no way to identify any of them. Shirabe's youngest daughter, however, found a piece of half-burnt cloth on which the name Hiroharu was read. It belonged to the second son of Professor Shirabe. No other remnant was found.

His oldest son, Seiichi, was in an arms factory in Ohashi, 1.2 kilometers from the hypocenter, when the bomb exploded. He had burns over his head, back and arms, but was able to walk to his home. The relief of his family turned to grief because he died one week later, although the burns were limited to one third of his body surface. The death of his second son was another heavy blow to the Professor, who nearly collapsed, without any hope or energy left in him.

Nevertheless, he went to see the sick victims whenever he was asked, disregarding the distance and his fatigue. One day he went a long way to attend a staff meeting of the medical school. When he came home, his strength was gone. The next morning he found many red spots on his arms and thighs. Subcutaneous hemorrhage, a sign of post-radiation leukemia, started. He realized that he could no longer escape the fate which took the life of the Dean and his two sons. General malaise and loss of appetite progressed. He had no strength to speak.

He could not sleep at night, thinking of the future of his wife and three daughters after his death. This state of helplessness and anxiety lasted one week. Then he noticed the change of his skin color, from red to purple and from purple to yellow. White cell count increased to the normal range. It was at this stage that a medical student came and found a bottle of alcohol. He advised Professor Shirabe to drink a glass of ethyl alcohol mixed with a ten percent glucose solution. It tasted good. Professor Shirabe emptied the glass and it warmed his body. After that, he took a glass of alcohol every morning and evening. He felt his strength coming back to him, although he did not know whether the drink helped him or not.

Professor Shirabe later made the following observations to Professor Yasuo Yoshizawa of Tokyo University in an interview:

"Those who were exposed to the fatal dose of radiation at the beginning had no chance of survival. Those who received a mild dose of radiation survived without any problem. It was the people in between whose survival depended on the treatment they received after exposure to a moderate amount of radiation. Some survived and others died. In regard to the distance, all cases within a radius of one kilometer were grave. Mortality was nearly 100 percent. No one died outside of the three kilometer radius. Moderate cases were those who were exposed at a distance of between one and three kilometers. The closer the distance, the higher was the death rate. In this group, the amount of radiation absorbed determined the outcome, and the dose of radiation always depended on the location and posture of the exposed individuals and on the type and structure of the shelter or building if there was any. Accurate measurement of the dose of radiation was impossible. We could only guess. According to Dr. Nishimori, Professor of Pathology of our school, one half of those who received 400rem of radiation would die within two months. The dose of gamma-rays at a distance of 1.2 kilometers was 391rem."

Mrs. Koyano and Professor Shirabe were exposed at the same distance of 700 meters from the hypocenter, but the former died and the latter survived. It was a difference in fate, but also it was a difference in dosage. Individual resistance and physical strength might influence the outcome. My classmate Mochizuki went home carrying the remains of his wife Michiko, who died near the place where Mrs. Nagai was also killed. Afterward, all of his hair fell out. But he did not die.

The peak of death came ten days after the bomb and again fifteen or sixteen days after the bomb, as observed at the Omura Navy Hospital and at the Kawatana Hospital, both in Nagasaki Prefecture.

*"May the soul of the dead rest in peace in the Grace of our Lord!"* Prayers for dying patients sounded at night in many different parts of the destroyed First Urakami Hospital building. I could not escape the smell of cremation in the hospital yard.

In a typical Urakami Catholic family such as Yamagami's, John, the oldest son, was killed in the arms factory, three-year-old

Peter died under the pressure of the ruined house. Four other brothers were pulled out of the debris by their mother, but died one after another, on the 11th and 18th of August and on the 21st and 23rd of September. The only ones left in the family were the parents, who were also exposed and injured but survived. Of all 12,000 Urakami Catholics 8,500 died, more than two-thirds. Drafted fathers came back to their empty Urakami homes and stood in sorrow on the burnt land where their families once lived together in happiness.

In the First Urakami Hospital, the staff and the helping hands worked hard trying to save as many as possible, but their efforts failed to save the victims of the devilish bomb. It was more than a month before the second wave of death subsided in the hospital.

Dr. Nagai gave mineral water to the patients and injected vitamin C and vitamin Bs. Treatment with liver and vegetables was also attempted. Dr. Akizuki gave the patients his "mineral nutrition" diet of brown rice and soybean soup daily. A little salt was added but no sugar was allowed. Pumpkins and eggplant were also his recommended foods. Some of them must have worked. The patients regained their strength and went home one after another. There remained only old tuberculosis patients who had been there before the bombing.

In September, I had diarrhea. I did not worry about it because I did not find petechiae in the skin. Dr. Akizuki, however, advised me:

"Why don't you take a rest for a while? We don't have many patients anymore."

He worried about me, because I was exposed to radiation at a closer distance than he was. There was a rumor that no grass would grow in Urakami for the next 75 years. I accepted his advice and took a trip to Southern Kyushu to see my old friend Masakuni Chiba who was graduated from the Doshisha Theological Seminary and became a minister of a local Protestant church in Miyazaki Prefecture.

# 4

# THE MEDICAL SCHOOL IN EXILE

The beauty of the Nichinan seashore was a contrast to Urakami ruined by the atomic bomb. I met Masakuni Chiba for the first time after five years of separation. He was glad that I had survived the bomb, and welcomed me with his wife Kazuko, a former kindergarten teacher. They asked me to speak at the church on Sunday. They also took me to Miyazaki, Aoshima, and the scenic coast of southeastern Kyushu. The time passed too soon. I had to go back to Nagasaki, keeping in mind all the beauty of the Southern ocean and rich greens of Miyazaki Prefecture.

I went back to the First Urakami Hospital because the Nagasaki Medical School was completely destroyed. Four professors survived the bomb, but all were sick except Professor Koyano. The majority of the medical students died and the surviving students went home and stayed home. I had no other choice.

Makurazaki typhoon on the 16th of September attacked and destroyed Nagasaki further, but it helped to remove the residual radioactive particles from the city. After the typhoon, the patients did not die any more. Dr. Akizuki regained his health. Miss Fukahori recovered from her injury and emaciation. The cool autumn air might have refreshed her. Brother Alcantara was released from his long internment since the beginning of the Pacific War in 1941. He came back to Urakami again as a Franciscan Brother. This muscular Canadian did not waste time. Immediately after his arrival, he started to remove the debris from the ruins of the hospital. He worked every day from early morning until late in the evening. In a short time he built a small, clean chapel and a neat residence for the staff and seminary students. He designed the new clinic building and kept working for it, encouraging us with his smile.

At the same time in September restoration of Nagasaki Medical School started in Omura, 30 kilometers north of Nagasaki. Rear Admiral Yasuyama of Omura Navy Hospital was a graduate of Nagasaki Medical School. He was shocked at the number and severity of injury of the atomic bomb victims transported to the hospital from Nagasaki on August 9. Many of them died before the treatment started. He ordered Lieutenant Commander Kiyoshi Hara, another graduate of Nagasaki Medical School, to do everything possible for the patients. The medical records and statistics of 758 patients were later reported by a young Navy Surgeon, Masao Shiozuki, as *A Survey of Atomic Bomb Casualties Treated in Omura Navy Hospital.*

Dr. Yasuyama wanted to see with his own eyes how badly the medical school hospital was damaged. He took a train to Nagasaki on September 24. At first he visited Professor Emeritus Kunitomo at his bed in Katafuchi, Nagasaki, and then went to Urakami. What he saw in Urakami on that day was later described in his book *A Record of the Atomic Bombing in Nagasaki.*:

"Not a single house remained in the valley and hills on both sides of the Urakami River. The color of the roads was brick-brown. The ruins of the houses left nothing but broken roof tiles. All trees were burnt to ashes. The soil of terraced rice fields was burnt to a dark brown color. I suppose no one in the nearby shelters had any chance of survival. As I imagined the scene and agony following the bombing, my body trembled in pain and sympathy."

When he approached the site of the medical school hospital, there came the nauseating smell of a dead horse on the slope below the main entrance. Nobody was in the hospital, which was completely burnt, leaving only the concrete walls of the building. It was nothing but a ruin. He realized that it was impossible to rebuild the medical school in Urakami in the near future.

When he returned to Omura in the evening, he was visited by Commander Dr. Dickson from the Fifth Fleet. He came to inspect the hospital before it was taken over by the U. S. Navy. After seeing 20 Navy patients and more than 500 severe cases of atomic disease, he concluded, "This hospital is well equipped and set up, but we will not take it over for our Navy. It should be used for the local patients. I believe this hospital should be used as a medical center of this area. All patients in the Shinkozen Emergency Medical Center should be moved here for better treatment. I will report my views to the Medical Director of the Fifth Fleet and he will report to General MacArthur."

When he had finished he stepped forward to the Japanese Commander, Dr. Tawara of Sasebo Navy Base, who attended Dr. Dickson. Dr. Tawara insisted that this hospital should be kept as a Japanese Navy hospital. Dr. Dickson said nothing.

What the U.S. Navy finally took over was the one remaining building of the Japanese Navy Hospital in Sasebo and a small regional subdivision in Isahaya City, between Nagasaki and Omura. Many beds were ordered for these two hospitals, and more than 1,200 wounded American soldiers were hospitalized. The U.S. Navy did not take over Omura Hospital, which had a capacity for 1,700 patients.

Dr. Yasuyama was excited by Dr. Dickson's statement and reported to the acting Dean, Professor Koyano. By September 26, three professors, one associate professor, six residents, six students, and three nurses arrived at Omura Hospital. Among them were Professors Shirabe, Kageura and Kitamura, Associate Professor Junnichiro Sato and a student named Hideo Tsuchiyama, who became the president of Nagasaki University forty years later. They were assigned to eight wings, and medical treatment and study started in Omura Hospital.

On the same evening, Major Dr. Warren came from Nagasaki to see Dr. Yasuyama asking for help in the study of the atomic bomb casualty research team headed by Captain Dr. Burnett, Professor of Pediatrics, St. Louis University. When Dr. Yasuyama explained to Dr. Warren his intention of using the hospital for the Nagasaki Medical School and how Professor Koyano was having difficulty at Sasebo to get permission to use the Omura Hospital as a teaching hospital, Dr. Warren agreed with him and promised to help him. When a group of U.S. Navy officers came from Sasebo to take over the hospital, Dr.Burnett's research team was already staying and working in the hospital. Therefore, confiscation was postponed. This research team investigated and studied with skillful efficiency, and also helped the treatment of the patients by providing penicillin and other needed medicines. If a patient died, Dr. Warren came from Nagasaki to do an autopsy. A cooperative meeting on

September 30 was attended by forty U.S. medical officers and twenty Japanese scholars. At this meeting Professor Koyano reported the enormous damage done to the Nagasaki Medical School and asked for help to transfer the Omura Hospital to the Medical School from the Navy.

On September 23, the Second Marine Division entered the harbor of Nagasaki. A few days later the 42nd Military Government Team set up headquarters near the pier. The only doctor in the government team was Captain Herbert W. Horne, Jr., who had studied at Harvard and Columbia universities. He felt deeply sorry for the devastation of the medical school,and proposed to the Governer of Nagasaki Prefecture and the Mayor of Nagasaki City to provide the Shinkozen primary school and the former army hospital in Nagasaki as affiliated hospitals to the medical school. Professor Shirabe told him that they were too small to be teaching hospitals of the medical school. Dr. Horne, Jr. agreed and wished to add the Omura Hospital.

He went to Omura and examined the hospital. At the end he told Dr. Yasuyama, "Omura Navy Hospital is a well-equipped hospital with large grounds and good buildings. This would be an ideal substitute for the destroyed Nagasaki Medical School Hospital. It is my responsiblity as an occupation army administrator to transfer this hospital to Nagasaki Medical School and make it the center of medical treatment and medical study in Nagasaki Prefecture."

He promised Dr. Yasuyama to send this recommendation to G.H.Q. On the 14th of October the Military Government in Nagasaki announced, "The Omura Navy Hospital should be transferred to Nagasaki Medical School and it will become the Medical Center of Western Kyushu. This decision has already been reported to the Commanding Office of General MacArthur." However, Captain Horne's negotiation with the Chief Surgeon of the Fifth Fleet, Dr. Young, was unsuccessful. Professor Koyano also went to Sasebo to meet Dr. Young, but was turned down.

Whenever an army doctor came to the First Urakami Hospital, I acted as an interpreter for Dr. Akizuki, because I had more experience in English conversation than Dr. Akizuki, who had studied German in High School. One day Captain Horne, Jr. came to the First Urakami Hospital and took a look at the hospital. Before he left the hospital, he told me, "I need a medical student like you who is good in English. Would you come with me and help us?"

I went with him to Dejima, to the empty army hospital which had been used as a training center for Japanese immigrants to Brazil before the war. It was located near the harbor, just below Kassui Mission School for Women, and one block from the customs house where the headquarters of the American Military Government were set up. Captain Horne, Jr. wanted to make this small hospital into a new medical center for the citizens as soon as possible. He named it "Blair General Hospital." No Japanese knew the source of the name but it had also a Japanese name, "Jikei Hospital." "Jikei" means "grace" in Japanese. The damaged interior was repaired and repainted.

My job was to make a list of a large stock of medicine and medical supplies stored in the warehouse standing along the pier opposite the hospital. The Japanese interpreter must have hesitated to translate the Japanese medical terms into English and classify them according to the type of the medicine. Every day I went to Dejima and worked with American officers. It was not an easy job, but I did my best. They were kind to me and offered me many nice things we needed, because they needed my help. My work was finished by the end of October, when rebuilding of the hospital was completed. The new hospital started on December 1, with Dr. Katsumi Takao as the Superintendent and Dr. Minoru Maeda as the chief surgeon. This Jikei Hospital was under the management of the Nagasaki Medical Association at first, but two years later it was transferred to the City and named Nagasaki Citizens' Hospital. Later, new wings and floors were added to the hospital and it has served the citizens of Nagasaki to this day.

The Shinkozen primary school was used as the outpatient clinic for the medical school, and the Omura Hospital for inpatients. I seldom attended the clinic and hospital, because I was too busy in Dejima. Occasionally I went to Omura from Nagasaki. It was another world, compared with Nagasaki. The Omura Hospital was intact because no bomb had been dropped during the war. The hospital was not crowded because many patients ran away from the hospital when the occupation by the U.S. forces was expected. The only patients who stayed were those with severe or chronic illness. A number of vacant wings were allowed for the use of students, who enjoyed the free space and a big bathroom. In the bath we appreciated our good luck, showing each other wounds and burn scars. On our way to Omura Station we walked through the potato fields and asked the farmers to sell us some of the crop they were harvesting. They did not accede to our eager request until they found out that we were hungry medical students. We spent all the money we had for the potatoes and pumpkins, because rations of rice did not reach us for months. I will never forget the sweet taste of the sweet potatoes we brought back to Nagasaki and Miss Hirakawa cooked for us at the Furumachi Church. She was not strong enough to travel in the crowded train carrying heavy sacks, but she gave us used kimonos or hand-tailored dresses to exchange for potatoes or pumpkins. She thanked us for our bartered products.

Professor Koyano was officially recognized as the Dean of Nagasaki Medical School by the Minister of Education, but there was no assurance that the seventeen professors who were killed would be replaced. In fact, there was a rumor that our medical school might be abolished. As a representative of all students, I was asked to appeal personally to Mr. Yoshinari Abe, the Minister of Education in Tokyo.

On my trip to Tokyo to see Mr. Abe I had great difficulty in finding his house because so much of the city lay in ruins. In fact by the end of the War at least half or more of the urban area of Tokyo had been destroyed by B29 bombers and other aircraft. In some areas the scorched earth was totally barren of homes; only concrete buildings remained to dot the landscape. It took several hours before I found him in his home after trying many labyrinths in the ruins of Tokyo. The Minister of Education listened to my petition in grave silence. He promised me at last,"I will do my best for the restoration of the Nagasaki Medical School." I do not know how much my petition helped the future of our school. I saw the miserable reality of our metropolis with my own eyes. How could I expect a speedy recovery of our school, which was completely destroyed by the atomic bomb? I left Tokyo with a heavy heart.

Our ties of friendship with classmates became stronger as a result of our common experience in the disaster. We often bathed together in the big bath pool of the Omura Hospital. We were a family sharing scarce food together. When Mochizuki, a bass singer, came back from Kagoshima with improved health, we formed a glee club and sang together familiar old songs. We enjoyed singing in our rooms or outdoors. It was an age when entertainment was scarce and our spirits were depressed. But as we sang we became brighter and happier. Emaciated Sasaki regained his weight by and by, and Mochizuki and Yamaguchi grew hair again.

Someone suggested choral singing on a downtown street in Nagasaki to raise funds for the war orphans and war widows. The atomic bomb left many orphans in Nagasaki, and the war robbed husbands of many wives. It was the hardest time for orphans and widows with children. Orphanages and settlements for widows suffered from lack of funds. That was why we made up our minds to sing on a downtown street corner to collect money for them.

It was the first Christmas after the war. Seven medical students stood in front of the Okamasa Department Store and sang many Christmas songs and asked for contributions "for orphans and widows." We were glad whenever pedestrians threw money into a box. It was our first experience of singing on a street, but we were rewarded. The money collected was presented to a settlement house in the city for widows who lost husbands in the war. Representing the widows, Mrs. Mochida accepted our donation and all the widows thanked us for our project. It made us happy too.

I was tired. I knew I had lost my strength. Was it delayed fatigue from my activities following the atomic bomb? It was hard for me to travel in a crowded train with a heavy sack on my back. Rations became rarer and rarer, fewer and fewer. In February, 1946 I noticed my body temperature was higher than normal. Miss Hirakawa saw the difficulty I had climbing the stairs to the second floor, and put me in bed on the main floor. When a doctor examined me, he found lesions of tuberculosis in my lung. I had to stay in bed.

I was a leader of our class after the war. Besides, I had to act as leader for all the medical students. Many reports and requests came to my bedside. I was happy to hear of the official re-opening of our school on February 20, 1946, but my pleasure was tempered by disappointment. Dr. Yasuyama had to retire from the navy and leave the hospital on March 19, when the hospital was transferred to the Ministry of Health and Welfare and a newly appointed director came to Omura to take over the hospital. Repeated petitions from Dr. Yasuyama and Dr. Hara could not change the situation. Negotiations by Dean Professor Koyano with the Ministry of Education and Ministry of Health and Welfare were in vain. Nothing could be done by the Minister of Education against the refusal of G.H.Q. on this issue. On April 15, Colonel Sams of G.H.Q. came to Omura and called us all into the auditorium. In front of us he ordered Dean Koyano to move out of Omura by the end of April and thereafter use the Isahaya Division of the Navy Hospital as the teaching hospital for the Nagasaki Medical School. We were very much disappointed, because the Isahaya Hospital is much smaller and less well equipped than the Omura Hospital, even though the distance from Nagasaki is shorter, only 30 minutes by train.

# 5

# ECCLESIA

Furumachi means “gold town” in Japanese. Furumachi church was located in this old section of Nagasaki, three kilometers from the epicenter. It survived the bombing, although its roof and walls needed repair. Every Sunday I performed my duty at Furumachi Church after the war as before, no matter how tired I was, except the first Sunday after the bomb. My duty was to speak on the Bible message at the Sunday morning service. It was not a sermon. I did not like to preach a sermon. After all, I was not qualified to preach in the church, because I was not an ordained minister. I was a layman speaking about the Bible in a pastor-less church. Therefore, I did not stand at the pulpit. I stood on the floor below the pulpit and spoke to a small audience. It was not a lecture. I commented on the selected message of the Bible and confessed my faith.

Furumachi Church had had no minister for two years. Elder members were supposed to take the place of the minister, but everyone was too busy and hesitated to speak on Sundays. That was why they welcomed a student who had once studied theology in Doshisha University, Kyoto. They were happy to keep me in the vacant parsonage and let me speak on Sunday mornings.

However, the situation changed after the War. People did not work on Sunday any more. Those who had neglected church to avoid the suspicion of the police and public came back to church again after the end of the war. Those who heard of rich gifts to the church from American soldiers and overseas Christians approached the church, hoping for some benefits. They were called "Rice Christians." The number of people attending the Sunday service increased as the ration of rice decreased. The church wanted a regular pastor, and pastors who returned from the army needed positions in the church.

As I anticipated, one day in March a presbyter told me: "An ordained minister is coming to our church on the first of May. Please leave the parsonage by the end of April."

At that time in the parsonage, there lived four persons besides me: Miss Hirakawa, her niece Keiko, a church member who came back from Navy service, and Osamu Mori, who was my classmate in Doshisha and had come back from Qingdao, China, to apply to a medical school as I had. All had to find other places to live. It was sad to be separated from each other after living together in the same house. Miss Hirakawa had lived there since Pastor Yukichi Sonoda, her brother-in-law, moved to a local church in the center of Kyushu in May, 1944. As a deaconess she stayed in the parsonage and had to take care of me. The two of us lived during the hardest time of the war helping each other. In the true sense, we were "comrades" who fought together for the church in wartime and survived the atomic bomb. They said that survivors of the atomic bomb would not live long. How long would we live? Five or ten years? Probably I would die first because I was exposed at a closer distance than Miss Hirakawa. But she was not healthy. She often complained of fever and headache.

In spite of her physical weakness, she took good care of me. The church offered me a place to stay, but no payment for my service to the church. The church could not afford to, I suppose. It was Miss Hirakawa who supplied me with meals in the days of food shortage. I thought all expenses were paid by the church, but I found out afterwards that she paid for everything out of her small income from sewing. I owe so much to her generosity, which was near to sacrifice. But all came to an end.

I was considering going back to my father's house. Then one morning Miss Hirakawa handed me a small piece of paper at the porch before I left for school. I read the paper while I was walking. It said, "I want to be at your service forever."

Did it mean that she wanted to live with me even after we left Furumachi Church? No word of "marriage" was mentioned in the note, but what else could it mean? This was nothing but a proposal of marriage. What should I do?

I had had a few proposals of marriage since I became a medical student. With few exceptions, young men of marriageable age had been drafted to the army. Students, particularly medical students, were looked at as good bridegroom candidates. Some potential brides were recommended by my brother or my friends. Every time I declined. I told myself not to marry anyone until the war ended, because I saw a number of young widows who had lost their husbands in the war. Only once, however, I agreed reluctantly to meet a candidate for engagement, because it was Muneo Araki, my old friend, who recommended a young lady.

When I arrived at his home, the mother of the girl came to the porch to welcome me, and proudly listed the names of her relatives and friends in high society. I was disappointed and ran out of the house without meeting her daughter, because I knew that a daughter reflects her mother much more than a mother reflects her daughter. I saw no need of seeing her daughter because I had no intention of living with this woman. I would hurt the girl if I refused her after I met her. It would be better not to see her. But Araki was upset, and ran after me and begged me to see her once as he had planned. He said, "It's a marvelous chance for you. They would build a new house in Urakami for you, and will finance your study abroad."

I refused to go back and went home, though I felt sorry for him and his mother who arranged this chance for me. If I had accepted their deal and lived in a new home in Urakami, I might have lost my life in Urakami on the ninth of August.

I had never thought of marrying Miwa Hirakawa before. I did not pay much attention to her. She was older than I. She was born in 1906, the worst year of the horse according to Japanese superstition. I was born twelve years later in another year of the horse. But the big difference in our age did not matter. During the last one and a half years since I moved into the church, I could not live without her. She respected me, trusted me, and took good care of me. She devoted herself to me, because she thought I was indispensable to the church. It was the worst and the hardest time for any Japanese, especially in Nagasaki, and she stayed all the time as my faithful helper and comrade. I could live with her all my life. Above all, she has the most important virtue I expect of my wife-to-be. It is her faith. We have the same faith in Christ. We have learned the same view of life from the Bible. She wants to follow the teaching of Jesus,"Love thy neighbor," regardless of the cost to her. Faith is all we need. Other considerations are of secondary importance. She trusts God and she trusts me. She trusted this poor medical student and served me as if she was serving God through her service to me. I knew she was the kind of woman who would not hesitate to sacrifice her life for me. Why should I hesitate to marry her?

Instead of going to school, I went to the home of Mr. Kenji Masuda, a presbyter of Furumachi Church. Sitting in front of Mr. and Mrs. Masuda, I told them, "I want to marry Miss Hirakawa. Please, tell me your opinion."

As a Calvinist, Mr. Masuda looked serious and meditated in silence. But Mrs. Masuda gave me her prompt answer with a happy smile, "I am glad to hear that. I am all for you." Then Mr. and Mrs. Masuda promised to play the role of marriage arranger for us.

When I returned to my father's house and told him my intention, he had no objection, but commented, "If you think it's right, marry her. But are you sure you won't regret it in the future when you study abroad ?"

That was all he said. He had already been introduced to Miss Hirakawa at the last Christmas celebration after he attended the Christmas service for the first time in his life. His twin granddaughters had been invited to the parsonage in turn and enjoyed its hospitality. He would have been happier if he had known that Miss Hirakawa was born and lived in Oita Prefecture where he was born, but her home village was surrounded by mountains and quite far from his home village on the eastern coast of Kyushu Island. I found out this fact after we were married.

I went back to the parsonage and told Miss Hirakawa the result of my consultation. She buried her face in my chest. I should call her Miwa from now on. Before long she began making her wedding dress from a kimono her mother gave her before she died.

We were married at Furumachi Church on the Emperor's Birthday, a holiday, April 29, 1946. It was a simple wedding. My father stood behind me in his formal Japanese kimono. He was uneasy because this was his first experience of a Christian wedding in a church. After the service he congratulated us, saying, "A Christian wedding is not bad. I liked it." He must have been impressed by our pledge, "Whether we are rich or poor, whether we are well or ill...we promise to live together and love each other all the time, forever!"

After the ceremony, we gathered in a small upstairs room of the church to have a feast of celebration. All we had on the table of our "feast" were cups of tea and small pieces of potato cake, and nothing else. Yet I remember no other feast as being so rich and so happy. No more than thirty guests, my classmates and church members. No celebrity or formal guest. The only relatives of Miwa present were her younger sister and three nieces. It was such an informal and friendly gathering. Everyone recalled the time of hardship we shared together, and congratulated us on our good luck and present happiness. We sang many hymns together. Our glee club sang in chorus, much better than we did downtown at Christmas time. At the end of the feast I stood up and announced:

"This wedding was the dedication of a new ecclesia. I believe that a Christian home should be an ecclesia-in-home. The Greek word 'ecclesia' means 'those who were called out.' It was translated as 'church' in English, but any gathering of people with the same faith is an ecclesia. No church building is required in ecclesia. Sometimes the building and the system create not only formalism, but also illusion and confusion. An ecclesia was, and should be, a home of brothers and sisters of the same faith. It is sad that Christian churches now lack the homely atmosphere of a family, when they became too big and too formal. I hope that our new home will become a new 'ecclesia-in-home,' bound by faith and love. We welcome you to our new ecclesia any time."

We had no honeymoon. Soon after the wedding we moved to our rooms in the house of Mrs. Ueno, who kindly allowed us to use a section of her house standing on a hill looking over the downtown of Nagasaki. Mrs Ueno was an elder of Furumachi Church, and her husband was a kind gentleman. They helped us make a small but comfortable place to live.

Visitors had to walk up long stone steps from Maruyama Street. Yet many of our friends came to visit us and enjoyed our small ecclesia-in-home. I felt sorry for my father, who visited us from the other end of the city and climbed up the long steps, nearly two hundred he counted, stopping once or twice for rest on the way. He was delighted with Miwa's hospitality, and praised her as "the best bride in three worlds."

My classmates came to discuss in secret many problems in the school. There had been constant trouble. The medical school had to move from Omura to Isahaya. Old and new professors disagreed on every plan for the future. Student unions were becoming too radical at the national level. In our own medical school, students were against each other, and radicals were demanding general strikes. As the general secretary of our student union, I had to moderate the radicalism of some students in order to assure the future of our school. I had a team of several good assistants, old glee club members. My home was often used as secret headquarters to avoid news reporters who tried to find out our strategy and plans. We worked hard to build harmony in the school, among professors and among students. We also worked to distribute scarce textbooks to students without unfairness. Mochizuki succeeded in obtaining a ton of beans from a farmers' union for the students in the dormitory, to save them from starvation. He was not always lucky. His only shoes disappeared from our porch one day while he was staying in our home. People were poor and hungry. Some of Miwa's best kimonos also disappeared from our new home.

In the autumn, I started a Bible study meeting at our ecclesia-in-home. A small group of Christian friends attended this Bible class at home on Sunday. The text was the first letter of St. Paul to the Corinthian ecclesia. I translated the Greek text into plain Japanese. The climax was the 13th chapter.

*Even though I speak in human and angelic language and have no love, I am as noisy brass or a clashing cymbal. And although I have the prophetic gift and see through every secret and through all that may be known, and have sufficient faith for the removal of mountains, but I have no love, I am nothing. And though I give all my belongings to feed the hungry and surrender my body to be burned, but I have no love, I am not in the least benefited. Love endures long and is kind; love is not jealous; love is not out for display; it is not conceited or unmannerly; it is neither self-seeking nor irritable, nor does it take account of a wrong that is suffered. It takes no pleasure in injustice, but sides happily with truth. It bears everything in silence, has unquenchable faith, hopes under all circumstances, endures without limit. Love never fails.... There remain then, faith, hope, love, these three; but the greatest of these is love. (Berkeley version)*

# 6

# ENGLISH CLASS

The medical school hospital in Isahaya started in May, 1946. This former branch of Omura Navy Hospital had deteriorated after the war. Cleaning and repair work were needed. A group of medical students responded to the call of Hatano, my classmate. They went there and worked hard every day to get ready for the opening of a new teaching hospital.

The medical college attached to Nagasaki Medical School in wartime was abolished. Three students who had been studying medicine in Manchuria until the end of the war were added to our class. Yet the number of our classmates was only 47. We had expected to graduate from the medical school in three and a half years of constant study without vacations. But now we had to stay for four full years before graduation.

Isahaya Hospital was a textile factory before the war started. The building was not large enough for a hospital, in sharp contrast to the spacious Omura Hospital. The patients in Shinkozen primary school hesitated to move to Isahaya Hospital because of the long distance from Nagasaki and the hospital's poor set-up. They preferred the newly-built Blair General Hospital in Nagasaki. Isahaya Hospital could not get enough patients for clinical teaching. Professors could not find a case to present at the clinical lecture. The chance for post mortem autopsy was nearly zero. The new students of 1946 had to study anatomy without a human corpse to dissect. Time was wasted in Isahaya. The third-year and fourth-year students were expected to listen to the clinical presentation in Isahaya after attending the outpatient clinic in Nagasaki. But the one-hour train trip to Isahaya from Nagasaki was not easy during the post-war period. After arrival at Isahaya we were often disappointed by the announcement "No clinical lecture this afternoon." We spent more time in food hunting and part-time jobs than in school.

I needed a source of income, too. No money came from anybody to support me. My oldest brother and his family in Nanjing were kept in a camp since the surrender of the Japanese army. My sister-in-law died in the camp after delivering a child. My brother returned to Nagasaki with his boy and his new baby. He could not find a job in Nagasaki and sold my father's belongings one after another to buy food for his family of two boys and two girls. A kind neighbor recommended a second wife for him, but she did not stay longer than one week. My brother disappeared with his older son, leaving the baby boy and two daughters. My father sent the three children to their mother's relatives, and he remained in his house alone. I had no income to help my father. Miwa supported me. She made dresses out of her old kimonos and sold them on the street. Sometimes I exchanged them for food. Rice was a rare luxury. Our scanty daily food consisted of potatoes and pumpkins. A surprising exception was a big gift of lobsters from Captain Horne, Jr. He gave them to us because he could not consume such a big seafood gift. In May and June we had the luxury of eating delicious plumlike loquats everyday, because famous Mogi loquats were sold cheap in Nagasaki that year due to paralyzed transportation to other cities in Japan. They disappeared, however, by the end of June.

In desperate financial straits, I turned to teaching English as a source of income, since young Japanese wanted to learn English conversation in post-war Japan, occupied by the U. S. Army. During the war, English had been an enemy language and consequently had not been taught in Japanese schools. Under the occupation, however, one needed a knowledge of English to find a good job in Japan. As a result, English conversation study flourished. NHK's new English Conversation Program was the most popular program among young people who were looking for a job or chocolate. One day I got the idea of starting an English conversation class in Isahaya. Rev. Aoyama had already started an English conversation school in Nagasaki and it was growing rapidly. But there was no English conversation class in Isahaya. I saw that the Isahaya Church could be a good place for the class. I visited Mr. Nishiyama, an elder of the Isahaya Church and also the principal of a small private school for women in Isahaya, and asked for his help. He agreed, and we started the "Isahaya English

Conversation Class" in the church twice a week in the evening.

The teaching members were medical students, two classmates and myself. Young people rushed in when the class started. As head of the staff, I taught English conversation from a textbook I had prepared. My elaborate study of English in my school days paid off, financially helping us. The attending students seemed as happy as I was.

But disappointment came before long. The number of students attending decreased every time. The early enthusiasm of the young people gradually died down. They might have been disappointed because they saw only young, inexperienced Japanese teachers. We could not continue the class with such a small enrollment. We gave up at last, and closed the class at the end of August, 1946. Afterwards we missed the fun of singing English songs together.

Miss Momoe Tomonaga, one of the old Furumachi Church members, was married to another member of the church, Otohiko Nobeta, while I was in Manchuria, and lived in Seoul until the end of the War. They came back to Nagasaki with their children in October, 1945 and attended Furumachi Church on Sundays. They invited us poor medical students to their one-room home and treated us with their generous hearts and meager meals during the hardest time. Shortly before we were married, Mr. Nobeta was appointed as the head of a branch of the Eighteenth Bank and they moved to Fukahori, a suburban town outside of Nagasaki.

It was in the spring of 1947 when I learned of the critical condition of their nine-year-old son. It was a result of indigestion due to infection. A medical student was helpless to save the child without the new antibiotic drugs not yet available in our defeated country. Tsugu-hiko died on April 24, 1947. I could not hold back the tears as I sang a hymn with his parents and his sister Motoko, looking at his remains:

*Tears fall on my sleeve when I try to call back my child*
*Who was dearer than gold or diamond,but frail as the dew on a leaf.*
*I shall, however, leave him in the hand of Jesus, who told us;*
*Death is not the end of life. It's the beginning of an eternal life.*
*Oh, to Jesus, I leave my beloved soul, to Jesus, our Lord.*

*(Sumi Kega 1929, composed by Seigi Abe)*

It was not only children who lost their strength of life and suffered hardship. Rations of rice stopped for four months. Some of the medical students who occupied a wing of the ruined hospital building in Urakami suffered so severely from the food shortage that they could not get out of their beds. Mochizuki tried hard to get beans from the farmers' union in Isahaya and brought them to Nagasaki with the help of others to make soup for the hungry dormitory students. Final examinations for the undergraduates were often postponed because so many students were ill. I failed my final tests in ophthalmology and dermatology. Professor Hirose, the new professor of ophthalmology who succeeded to the post of the late Professor Yamane, told me cynically at the test, "I don't remember if I saw you in my class."

The new professor of dermatology, Professor Seiichi Kitamura, did not forgive my early morning visit. I caught him at his home and asked him to stand on the side of our Dean Koyano instead of siding with Professor Hasegawa, who opposed the Dean's policy. As I expected, I failed in these two subjects and had to take re-examinations. By this time, Professors Hirose and Kitamura must have thought that they had punished me enough. They granted me the minimum grade needed for graduation. During the summer vacation before graduation, I worked at the private clinic of Dr.Toshio Kobayashi, whom I respected not only as a dermatologist but also as a talented painter. He taught me a little more about dermatology to fill the gaps in my knowledge.

Miwa became pregnant but had a miscarriage. Insufficient food supply and the long flight of stone steps to reach our home on the hill were too much for her. I looked for a hospital for my internship in some other town to secure a better food supply for Miwa's health. It was too bad in Nagasaki. I wanted to see the former Navy Hospital in Ureshino, Saga Prefecture, north of Omura.

To reach Ureshino, one has to take a train to Sonogi Station north of Omura, and then take a bus ride over a hill to Ureshino. Beyond the pass on the hill you find rich tea fields with green leaves. While you are marveling at the Arcadian beauty of this valley, you reach Ureshino, an old hot spring town. The town was still peaceful and quiet in 1947, with the old Japanese style inns around the stream. Away from the stream stood a stately hotel named Shinsenkaku. The old Navy Hospital was located behind the hotel. It was a big hospital which took care of many sick navy sailors and officers during wartime and many casualties of the atomic bomb in Nagasaki. This hospital, with more than 500 beds, stood in front of a mountain and was equipped with a good, hot spring bath. It looked like paradise to the eyes of visitors from the cities torn by air raids.

Most of the staff were former navy doctors, but the doctor I wanted to meet was an alumnus of our medical school, Dr. Kiichiro Okazaki, who came to this hospital as the Assistant Director from his previous position at Saga Sanatorium. He welcomed me with his warm smile and guided me through the hospital. At noon, he kindly invited me to his home for lunch. It was an official residence just outside the hospital. Mrs. Okazaki was a tall, graceful lady. She was the daughter of a store owner in Nagasaki. A small girl of around the age of three was hanging behind her, trying to see me. The girl dropped her eyes as soon as her eyes met mine, and she hid behind her mother.

While I was explaining to Dr. Okazaki my wish to take my internship in Ureshino Hospital, I noticed on his shelf a row of books by the late Takeshi Fujii, a famous disciple of Kanzo Uchimura who wrote *How I Became a Christian.* I told myself that Dr. Okazaki must be a good teacher for me, because he was a reader of Fujii's books. I decided on the spot to take my internship with Dr. Okazaki. Fujii's books made me decide. I was glad that I had found the right hospital for me.

The Nagasaki Medical School graduation was held in Isahaya Hospital one day in September, 1947. I was impressed by the speech of the Director of the medical school hospital, Professor Yasushi Mitani:

"I asked an American doctor in the occupation army for his definition of democracy. 'A sense of duty, and care for others' was his answer. As the new graduates of our medical school, keep in your mind these key words: A sense of duty, and care for others."

Representing all new graduates, as I had represented my class throughout the past four years, I expressed my thanks to our professors. At the end of my speech I added,

"We had 80 classmates when we started our study of medicine. Only half of them are graduating today. It makes us sad that the other half of our classmates could not share the joy with us, because they were killed by the atomic bomb. We have the determination now to work twicc as hard as other doctors to fulfill the unfinished wish of our deceased classmates by serving the people and treating their illness."

After the graduation ceremony we moved to Nagasaki to have our photograph taken with the professors in front of the ruined hospital building where we experienced the tragedy of the atomic bomb.

# 7

# URESHINO HOSPITAL

Four interns reported to Ureshino Hospital on October 1, 1947. They were Taizo Mitsutake and Sukehiko Yoshida, graduates of Kyushu University, and Hideo Kuriaki and I, graduates of Nagasaki Medical School. We were given rooms in a dormitory for single doctors. A tall, old woman took care of us in the dormitory. Next to our dormitory there was a hot spring hotel called Ureshino-kan. In front of our building stretched tea fields. The environment was not bad. I was satisfied with my temporary residence in Ureshino, although I was looking for a house where Miwa and I could live together.

Four interns were assigned to different departments in the hospital. We shifted every two to three months to another department. But four interns were not enough for this large hospital, which was three times larger than the temporary medical school hospital in Isahaya. We were quite busy, but learned much more than we would have in the medical school hospital. In the department of surgery, I assisted in nearly every operation. The chief surgeon, Dr. Shoichi Karazawa, was a hilarious man. He joked in the surgical theater to relax tense assistants. When I was assisting a young surgeon in carotid gland surgery, he cut the carotid artery by mistake. Red blood splashed and I was upset. The surgeon said, "Don't worry." But his hands were trembling. I trembled too, until Dr. Karazawa came in and managed to stop the bleeding.

I was interested in surgery of the lung. In those days, thoracoplasty was a popular surgery for pulmonary tuberculosis. Its aim was to collapse the involved lung by resecting a number of the upper ribs from the back. Another method to collapse the lung was to inject air into the pleural space through the chest. But there were disadvantages; the air must be injected every week to supplement the absorbed air, because the pressure of the decreased air is not sufficient to compress the cavity. Therefore, thoracoplasty, a surgery to compress the pulmonary lesion, was performed every week for the patients with larger cavities, and I gained confidence in my skill. Around this time a new compression technique using plastic balls was introduced by Professor Chuzo Nagaishi of Kyoto University. Dr. Karazawa adopted the technique and operated on many cases. I learned this new procedure before long.

Dr. Naoto Sugioka was an orthopedic surgeon with a character quite different from Dr. Karazawa's. He was a man of tight lips and robust build. When we were scrubbing our fingers with a brush and disinfectant, Dr. Sugioka approached us with a glass containing agar medium and printed our fingertips on the agar to check for the presence of any remaining bacteria. His test made us cautious about disinfection of our fingers before surgical operations. He was successful in his method of teaching us the aseptic technique.

Living quarters consisting of one room in a local law office were provided for me by the kind arrangement of Mr.Ikeda, my old acquaintance in Saga. Miwa was happy to move from Nagasaki to our new home in Ureshino.We carried everything we could carry with us on the train and then onto the bus at Sonogi. The charcoal bus stopped several times on the hilly road. Each time the passengers were requested to step out and push the bus from behind. When we arrived at Ureshino and unloaded my books and Miwa's sewing machine, our one-room home left little space for us to lie down. Nevertheless, it was our own sweet home.

Fortunately we soon found an old house to rent. Owned by a former Mayor of Ureshino, it was located only five minutes' walk from the hospital. The news of our new home brought many guests to Ureshino, including my old classmates and Miwa's relatives. They all enjoyed Ureshino and our country house. We had little money but plenty of hospitality. It was hard on Miwa, who often had to go to a pawn shop for money.

My father visited us in Ureshino for the first time on January 23, 1948. He was no longer in Nagasaki. He was living with his second son, my brother in Saga City, Saga Prefecture, north of Nagasaki Prefecture. He visited us in Ureshino, coming from Saga with my sister-in-law. My father appreciated Miwa's kind care. He joined us in our morning service and tried to sing the hymn with us, reading the words in the hymn book through his glasses:

*I remember now in shame how I left my father's house,*
*Chasing after the dream in vain, looking for joy in wine.*
*Ending in the pasture of swine, lying in the hut of grass.*
*The cold wind of the ruthless world tears my cloth and aching heart.*
*The dew of night reminds me of the tender love of my father I miss*
*Let me bring my soul to home, the home of the father I dearly love.*
*(Kirisutokyo Seikashu, 1895)*

My sister-in-law thanked God in prayer with tears in her eyes. At the end, my father saluted the Bible and told us, "I must learn how to thank Him, too."

During the five days of his stay in our house, he read with us five chapters of the New Testament: Luke 15, Matthew 5, 6, Luke 6, and First Corinthians 13. He appreciated everything including the hot spring spa,and went back to Saga, promising us a second visit.

A new Director of Ureshino Hospital came in late January, 1947. It was Professor Koyano, who had been the Dean of Nagasaki Medical School since the end of the war. His arrival made me happy. It was already two and a half years since we were bombed in the same room. He looked well. He had changed from a serious professor to an amiable gentleman. He attended our Bible study meeting every Tuesday evening at Mr. Nakamura's home. I used to be his student listening to his lectures on surgery, and now I spoke about the Bible in front of him. He would not sit on the upper seat. I was uneasy and hesitated, but he insisted, "You are the speaker at this meeting. This is right." He listened to me on the lower seat with the others.

In the hospital, my position was the opposite. I was in the lowest rank of the staff, and had to run around the hospital in a hurry. I was relieved when my term in surgery ended, because it was the busiest department. The next assignment was the department of internal medicine where I enjoyed working with Dr. Okazaki. He taught me about patients and their diseases kindly, keeping his smile all the time. His gentle attitude to the patients made him a popular physician in the hospital.

When I moved to the ophthalmology department, Dr. Ogasawara trusted me and let me see and treat the patients freely. He did not know that I had failed the final examination in ophthalmology at school. Neither did I know that his wife was a daughter of Professor Emeritus Kunitomo. Mrs.Ogasawara was a charming lady, particularly when she appeared from the green tea field wearing a bright red sash on her dark blue kimono and walked down to our house.

Dr. Daisuke Katamine came to Ureshino Hospital as a new chief of the department of dermatology and urology. He was not only an older graduate of Nagasaki Medical School but also a graduate of Saga High School, as I am. His father knew my father well because he was born in Oita Prefecture, as my father was, and they both belonged to the same Buddhist temple, called Koeiji. Dermatology was no longer a difficult subject for me, since I had been trained in the clinic of Dr. Kobayashi in the summer after I failed the final test on dermatology. Dr. Katamine treated me as a friend rather than an intern. We often ate together the meals prepared by the head nurse.

I found, however, a best friend in Dr. Masayoshi Satomi, a pediatrician. He was born in Shanghai, China. After the war he and his family came to Ureshino, where Mrs. Satomi had been born. They lived in an old warehouse with their four sons. Dr. Satomi was small and thin but he worked hard. He thought scientifically as a scholar but his attitude was kind, not only to the patients but also to me. One night we were both on duty and slept in the same room in the hospital. Lying on the beds, we talked about ourselves and our experiences in the past. Since then, we have been good friends. He attended our Bible study meeting and listened to my interpretation. It was not easy for me to speak in the presence of this scholar of pediatrics.

I had to prepare for the national test of physicians to get my medical licence. It was difficult for us to find time to read books in this hospital with more than 500 beds and only four interns. We had, however, plenty of experience in all fields of medicine. It was an ideal hospital to acquire clinical knowledge and skill. This was our advantage. I made hundreds of cards, picking up the necessary information from the textbooks, and memorized the notes between the busy assignments. There was no department of psychiatry in

Ureshino Hospital. To compensaate for this lack, we had to study for one week in a national hospital for mental diseases in Mitagawa, in the same Prefecture.

I took the national test in October, 1948 at Nagasaki University School of Commerce, which was not damaged by the atomic bomb because the building was protected by a hill between the bomb and the school in the eastern end of the city. I was thinking of asking my father to live with us after I passed this test and earned a salary from the hospital.

My father looked healthy when he came to Ureshino for the second time in April. He did not waste time. He made zori, Japanese straw sandals, and left them for us.

When my brother came to Ureshino he said to me, "Lend me a Bible with big print. Father wants to read it."

I happened to have a large Japanese Bible printed in the United States. I gave it to my brother. Later in a letter from my sister-in-law she wrote that my father started to read the Bible from Genesis. When I visited him in the summer, he was reading the Bible in his room on the second floor. The afternoon sunlight was bright on the open page.

"You see. This is his daily routine," my brother said and laughed. I looked at the thick pages of the Bible and thought of the length of his remaining days.

"My body doesn't work any more, but my brain does," my father laughed. In fact, he was taking care of the vegetable garden. He gave me his masterpiece, a big pumpkin, as a present to Miwa. He also washed his own underwear and worked to keep the house clean, perhaps because I told him once, "It would be good for your health, if you'd work on something you can do, rather than sitting still all day. It would be appreciated by the family, too."

I do not know if he followed my advice or not. He was a hard working man by nature. He did not waste his time in any game. He despised idleness. But the heat of this summer was too much for him. Edema was visible on his eyelids and legs. He became weaker and stumbled often. Injured wounds did not heal well. Bedsores bothered him and his difficulty with urination bothered the family.

One day in December I told myself that I should bring my father to Ureshino Hospital for check-up and treatment before it was too late. I planned to go to Saga on Saturday, but I was busy that day. It was the next Saturday when my brother phoned me from Saga, telling me that my father could not move any more. I hurried to Saga immediately.

The face of my father was entirely different from what I had seen the last time. I saw his time of death approaching. He was mentally confused. Large, necrotic bedsores were on both sides of his waist. I injected glucose solution into a vein, and treated the bedsores. He thanked me each time. He did not want to call a physician until I came. After my treatment, he started to sleep as if he were content. He had not been able to sleep the previous night, but he slept well this time. The next morning he looked better. He was in a better mood when he opened his eyes. But he had hallucinations, and his speech was not clear. He tried to tell me to be good to Miwa. He felt no pain as the result of uremia. I returned to Ureshino on Sunday afternoon.

Miwa went to Saga on Wednesday to visit my father, but he could not recognize her any more. He was in semi-coma. I wanted to visit him on Friday, but could not, because I had to give a speech in Ureshino Hospital on Friday. No telephone or telegram came on Friday. I hurried to Saga on Saturday, but my father was already dead when I arrived.

He was still lying in bed. My brother removed the cover from his face. There was the pale but peaceful face of my father. It had the expression of an infant. I cried and wept in deep sorrow.

I left him and went outdoors and looked up at the beautiful sky. I saw his peaceful face in the sky. Tears came down on my cheeks. I felt a lump coming to my throat.

He loved me more than any other son. He loved me far more than I loved him. He did not mind making sacrifices for me. He tried not to bother me. He wished to live with us, but he waited for the time when I could earn enough money to keep him with us. He was praying for the success of my national test. He did not want to disturb my work in the hospital even in his last days. The news of his critical condition came to me on Saturday. Our last visit was on Sunday. And the next Saturday morning his soul left this world quietly. The burial ceremony was on Sunday. Were the days of his last sickness and death all coincidental? I believe they were a revelation of his kind concern for me. He always yielded to my wish. Before the end of his 74 years of life, he yielded to my last and biggest wish. He read the whole Bible in his final year to understand the faith of his seventh son, and then died in peace. All his previous 73 years were preparation for this last year. He was born in a poor fisherman's family and fought against poverty all his life. For his seven children, he worked hard to earn money in the belief that money would solve our problems and make us happy. His expectations were not realized. He learned through sad experience that happiness is not in money or materials. He found true happiness apart from money or wealth in the last year when he lost all possessions and money. No more business wisdom was left in him. No strength of body was left for him. But he learned to appreciate the kindness of his sons and his daughters-in-law. He learned to be thankful for the grace and care of the creator unknown to him. We were amazed at the change in my father, from a dictator to a humble, tender father. My father had left nothing behind. His only small cloth bundle contained his memorabilia and three worn-out books on Buddha which he had read daily for many years since his young days. I remembered the words Professor Iwamoto once spoke to my father, "Your son reached to a sincere Christian faith because his father was a man of sincere faith in Buddhism."

I paid no respect to my father's faith. I was proud of being persecuted by my father. Now I realized that I had inherited from him a religious mind. His faith as a Buddhist drove me to my faith in Christ, and the tensions between us trained and deepened my faith. At the end, this single-minded, honest man read the whole Bible to understand the faith of his beloved son before he finished his 74 years of life.

One week later I received a telegraph that I had passed the national examination. It was December 25, 1948—a Christmas I can never forget.

# 8

# A TB DOCTOR

The Eleventh Wing of Ureshino Hospital was for tuberculosis patients. More than sixty patients were in this wing. The chief doctor was Dr. Tadashi Oba, and I was his new assistant. My dream had come to reality after ten years. As a doctor for tuberculosis patients I practised what I wanted to do.

First, I did not wear the white masks which all other doctors put on when they saw TB patients or walked in the wards. I had no reason to protect myself from tuberculosis bacilli because I had been a TB patient myself in the past. My reaction to the tuberculin test is negative, because I am immune to TB bacilli. Why should I protect myself from TB bacilli? TB patients with active lesions should wear masks when they meet non-patients to avoid contamination of others, but I am not a patient with an open cavity in the lung. Even if I had a cavity, there would be no need to wear a mask in this ward, because all patients have TB bacilli already. It is plain, simple logic. It is logical for tuberculin-negative doctors or nurses to wear masks in the ward to protect themselves. But it is a contradiction for a tuberculin-positive person to wear a mask as a protection. All the nurses in this wing are tuberculin-positive. They have no need to wear masks. It is all right if they want to wear masks, but I will not wear any mask.

The patients were surprised, and told each other, "The new young doctor examines the patients without a mask."

Some of them dared to ask me; "Doctor, why don't you wear a mask?" I answered them, "I myself was a TB patient. I am not afraid of TB bacilli. Why should I wear a mask?"

I was not sure if they understood me, but they were satisfied with my answer. They smiled as if they accepted me as one of them.

The tuberculosis patients were disliked and avoided as a dangerous source of contagion, not only by strangers but also by their own families, and doctors were no exception. Therefore, the patients in the Eleventh Ward looked at me with friendly eyes and trusted me.

Mild TB patients ate meals together in a large dining room in the middle of the wing. It saved the work of nurses, and helped patients to enjoy meals and conversation at mealtime. I proposed to eat with the patients once a week. This was something new for them, too. They were delighted. They enjoyed my company every week. They waited for the day with expectation. Flowers were arranged on the large table. Meals were ready for everyone. The patients came to the table hand in hand. Those who sat near my seat were envied. As the weekly dinner was repeated, we developed a kind of kinship. We understood each other more and more. I learned their feelings and problems. The patients did not hesitate to tell me about their wishes and desires. I told them frankly what I thought. It turned out to be a good chance for communication for all.

Every evening I walked around the ward and said "Good night" to every patient shortly before the lights in the rooms were turned off. My round was not welcomed by those who wanted to be alone with their lovers in the dark. Smokers could not hide from my eyes. My policy was to overlook smoking only once. If they smoked twice, ignoring my caution, they were discharged from the hospital for their violation of the hospital rule. No one objected to my policy, and as it happened, there was no need of enforcement of the rule in our hospital wards. Bedridden patients with advanced tuberculosis waited for my visit at night. It was an encouragement for them. It was also a chance for me to observe how the nurses behave at night without a supervisor. Nurses like to be complimented by a doctor when they are working hard at night.

Pneumothorax was still used as a non-surgical treatment for tuberculosis of the lung in 1949. On the day of pneumothorax, I had to inject air into the thorax of ten to twenty patients within a limited time. I invented a speedy way to facilitate the process. Two patients are placed on two beds. I sit close to one of them. I insert the long pneumothorax needle through the side of the chest into the narrow pleural space between the two pleural membranes inside the chest. Then starts the automatic injection of air by a pneumothorax machine, making a bubbling noise. While the machine is working, I approach the other bed and put the patient on his side. After disinfection of the skin, I wait for the end of air injection in the first patient. As soon as the last air is injected, I remove the needle, and put another new needle in the injector. Then the second injection starts on the second patient. By this time the third patient is already on the other bed, waiting for the disinfection of the skin. The same procedures follow, one after another, without wasting any second, as if an automatic machine were working. As a skilled, efficient technician, using this procedure I gave pneumothorax to as many as twenty patients in a few hours.

One morning, in the middle of my routine procedure, injecting and removing the pneumothorax needle, a patient behind me suddenly went into a state of shock. I looked at him in amazement. His face was pale. He was panting and could not speak, but his eyes were desperately asking for help. I did not know what I could do, and ordered the nurse to inform Dr. Oba, because I could not understand what happened. I saw he was suffering from a shortage of oxygen, for he was panting like a mad dog. With the help of a nurse I supplied him oxygen through an oxygen mask. I thought he would die, but gradually his dyspnea improved. Panting changed to regular but still fast respiration. The color in his face returned. For me it was my first shocking experience of spontaneous pneumothorax caused by a needle puncture of the surface of the lung. One lung collapsed but the other lung was intact and saved him, and the collapsed lung was re-inflated.

A few patients went home after being cured of their disease. Some left the hospital to continue bed-rest in their homes. But the majority of patients stayed in the hospital day after day, resting in bed. Bed-rest and good nutrition were the only treatment available for the TB patients until streptomycin was discovered. It was hard for physicians to see the gradual deterioration of their patients. As the physical strength weakens, the resistance of the patient against bacilli becomes lower and the lesion in the lung enlarges. It is a vicious circle. Eventually fever elevates and appetite is lost. Forced eating invites indigestion and diarrhea. Breathing becomes faster, and speaking rarer. At the end, with no strength to speak, there is only nodding and sad smiles in response to our words.

"Miss K is in critical condition, Doctor." A nurse told me in a hurry. I ran to her ward. Miss K was breathing in a hard way, but she tried to smile at me with her deep big eyes. I could not say a word. I took her hand and felt her pulse. Her pulse was weak and irregular. I pulled up a chair and sat at her bedside. I held her hand in mine and kept holding it. What else could I do? A poor helpless doctor. All I could do was to be near her. No relative was in the ward. Sudden change of her condition gave not enough time for her family to reach her. Or did they think of it as another alarm to which they had responded often but found that it was not the final one? Or were they afraid of the TB bacilli which fill the ward? I did not know. All I knew was that Miss K was facing death alone with none of her family or relatives at her bedside. The nurse left us. She was too busy to sit here and watch us. Here was a doctor, and she had to see other patients, for there were only two nurses for seventy patients at night. I was left alone in the midnight ward with a critical patient, Miss K. She was not just a patient. I knew each patient so well that I called them by their names. They were my close friends rather than my patients.

Miss K became quiet. She kept her eyes closed. Once in a while she opened her eyes to see if I was there, gave me a weak smile, and then closed her eyes with obvious satisfaction. Whenever her breathing became faster, my hand grip became tighter. Anxiety disappeared from her expression. She kept her hand in mine as if she trusted me and wanted me to stay with her. I stayed there, how long I don't know. At the end, she took a deep breath, stared at me with her big eyes, and then she expired. Her lips were still smiling. Tears ran out of my eyes. I knew she was trying to thank me.

All the patients in the TB wards loved me. I have never had any unpleasant experience there. I disliked none of them. We were a big family, a TB family. There was no wall separating us, the wall I felt at a TB ward in Saga many years ago. The only problem on the Eleventh Wing was the head nurse. She was bitter towards me because she thought I favored a young nurse who loved literature and was intelligent and efficient in her work. I suggested to Dr. Oba that he give this young nurse a supervisory position. The head nurse was jealous and hated me.

Suddenly I was given a new assignment. I was appointed as a doctor on the Ninth Wing. I had to leave the Eleventh Wing, which was to be changed to a ward for contagious diseases. All TB patients in the hospital were carried to the Ninth Wing. I was no longer an assistant doctor but a doctor in charge, responsible for the 50 patients on the second floor. This wing stood next to the hospital pond. From the second floor one could see the pond and the doctor's dormitory on the other side of the pond. The ward was a big, monotonous room with lines of beds. The patients lived in this big ward without trouble among them. In the middle of the long staircase there was placed a ceramic basin with flowers arranged beautifully in it. I was fascinated by its clean, simple arrangement. It was arranged every week by a male patient using different flowers each time. He told me that the style belonged to the Ohara School of flower arrangement. A white waterlily floating on the water of the basin was a beautiful contrast in this TB wing of the old Navy Hospital building. It consoled our hearts.

I was satisfied with my work as a TB doctor. I liked the hospital, too. The Director was Professor Emeritus Koyano, the former Dean of the medical school, and the Assistant Director was Dr. Okazaki. Both belonged to the Ureshino Bible Study Group with which I met once a week in the evening. Other, older colleagues were all nice and kind doctors from whom I learned many things. We four former interns welcomed new interns,who paid respect to us. We played volley ball games together and enjoyed dinner parties together.

One day I was called to the Director's room. Professor Koyano surprised me. He said, "Nagasaki City Hospital in Takenokubo wants you as a staff member. Would you go there and work for the city?"

I asked him why. He explained that the director of the hospital had visited Ureshino Hospital on another day to see our TB ward, and had been impressed by my report on the Ninth Wing. He told Professor Koyano his wish to have me as the chief of their new TB ward. They have residences for doctors near the hospital.

I hesitated for a moment. I was content in Ureshino. I had become used to the work and life in Ureshino Hospital. I had no complaint, no other ambition. Why should I go to Nagasaki, where the food situation was still worse than Ureshino? However,

Nagasaki is my home town. Takeno-kubo is in Urakami district, close to the old Nagasaki Medical School Hospital under reconstruction. The idea of starting a new TB wing was fascinating. It was an urgent need of the city to have a TB ward in the city hospital in this post-war period when tuberculosis was the No. 1 killer of Japanese. I was named as the best candidate for the job. I will follow the principle of John Wesley who wrote once:

*"Do not go where you want to go. Go to where you are needed most."*

I love Nagasaki also. It is my home town. I decided and answered Dr. Koyano, "Yes, I'll go to Takeno-kubo."

# 9

# TAKENO-KUBO

The name "Takeno-kubo" is not popular with the citizens of Nagasaki, because it reminds them of the crematory which is located in the Takeno-kubo section of Urakami. I remember my sad experience in the crematory,when I was ordered to light the fire to burn the body of my brother who died of acute peritonitis, because the one who was loved most by the deceased was supposed to start the fire. Next to this crematory stood a city hospital for contagious diseases. The official name is Nagasaki Hospital, but people called it the contagious hospital to avoid confusion with Nagasaki Citizens' Hospital, the new name of Blair General Hospital. Anyway, it was not a popular hospital in Nagasaki. Captain Horne ordered the city to admit TB patients to a wing of the hospital, because the number of patients with epidemic diseases decreased after the war in contrast to the increase of tuberculosis patients. I arrived at Nagasaki Hospital on the first day of September, 1949. The Director of the hospital was Dr. Yasuji Kawazoe, an old graduate of Nagasaki Medical School. Nearly all the old buildings had been destroyed by the atomic bomb. The new wooden buildings were built after the war. There remained in the yard the concrete foundations of the old buildings. At the end of the ruined yard, there stood two-story houses for doctors. They were small but new, with the advantage of being close to the hospital.

The wing for the TB patients was an old wooden building, standing on higher ground. From the window one could see the gate of the crematory. It would be an unpleasant view for patients. Behind the building is Mount Inasa. If one stands at the top of the hill, one has a view of the city of Nagasaki and harbor, but not from the window of this ward. It was not a good place for patients with chronic diseases, even though the location was convenient to send the dead to the crematory.

My experience in Ureshino Hospital contributed well to my new post. A few nurses came with me to this hospital from Ureshino, intending to continue their work with me. I designed an operating room for surgical treatment of pulmonary tuberculosis. As soon as a new surgical theater was completed in the building, I started to perform thoracoplasty, which aimed to compress the tuberculous lung lesion by resection of the overlying ribs. Dr. Masatoyo Yoshida, an internist, assisted me in the operation. There were some mishaps at the beginning, but the nurses and patients trusted me and helped me. I did my best to respond to their trust and respect. The food situation was still poor in Nagasaki. To supplement the shortage of food, patients and nurses worked together in the new vegetable garden near the wing. The crops made us happy. They were divided among patients evenly.

I had some acquaintances among the newly admitted patients. One of them was Kyoko, the wife of my old classmate at Nagasaki Middle School. Fortunately Kyoko was an early case of pulmonary tuberculosis and did not have to stay too long. Usually TB patients stayed longer. It is human nature that the longer they stayed, the closer we became. All patients became my good friends. Their improvement made me happy, and aggravation of the illness made me unhappy and depressed. If a patient died, I felt miserable and angry at my inability to save her. At times I wished to quit my job as a doctor.

A desperate doctor struggles hard
To find a way to save the sick,
Praying to find a way in vain.

He tries all kinds of medicine,
And infuses the blood into veins
As the anxious family watch him in vain.

The incapable doctor is in agony
To find a way to save the sick,
Praying to God to save him from death.

Writing such a poem did not cure my sick heart. I kept longing to study more somewhere. Then I happened to learn about the *GARIOA* Scholarship, which was renamed Fulbright scholarship after the end of occupation, a scholarship to provide the opportunity for young Japanese scholars and students to study in the United States. The fund came from the payment of the Japanese Government to the U.S. government for food supplies released to save Japanese people from starvation. I applied and received permission to take the examination.

The first part of the examination was a written test in Fukuoka to select the candidates from a large number of applicants. I passed the test and went to Tokyo to take the second test. Three testing members including two Americans asked me many questions in English. I tried to overcome my tension and answered all questions quietly. I was sure I had failed the test, because more than ten thousand people applied to get the chance of being included in the final selection of four hundred. It was an unexpected, happy surprise that I was selected as one of the *GARIOA* students for the year 1951. The majority of the selected students were residents of Tokyo. Only a few were from Kyushu. There were two medical doctors from Kyushu, a professor of pharmacology at Kurume Medical College and myself.

As the subject of my study I chose tuberculosis. Soon I was informed that I was accepted by the University of Michigan School of Public Health. I should have written "pulmonary surgery" instead of" tuberculosis" as my subject of study, because I wanted to learn the technique of pneumonectomy in order to remove tuberculous lesions of the lung. I knew there was an authority on pulmonary surgery at the University of Michigan, Professor Alexander, with whom I hoped I might get a chance to study lung surgery after finishing my study of public health. The University of Michigan is a good place for my study, I persuaded myself. The day of departure from Japan was set, Friday, July 13. The date did not sound nice, for the Last Supper was on Friday the thirteenth. But I decided not to think about it.

It was less than two years since I had started working at Nagasaki Hospital. The city thought it was too early to leave the hospital for a year's study abroad and that consequently, if I left, I should resign my post before leaving for the United States. But at the last moment, the city relented and gave me a leave of absence enabling me to return to my position and basic salary after my study abroad, as they also did with another employee who was selected as a *GARIOA* student. But they requested me to move out of the hospital residence, since they needed it for another doctor who was to substitute for me during my absence. Therefore, I had to look for a house. Houses were still few in Takeno-kubo, because nearly all buildings at this distance of one kilometer or less from the hypocenter were burnt down by the atomic bomb. The housing shortage was serious in Nagasaki. There was no choice but to build a house myself. Our deposit in the bank was far from sufficient for building a house, but we might have a chance to borrow money from the government at low interest to build our own house, if only we could find a suitable lot for sale.

I walked around Takeno-kubo area on the west side of the Urakami River, and looked for a place for our house until I found suitable land near the ruin of Chinzei High School. A doctor and his family were killed by the atomic bomb, and no one was living on the ruined land. The owner of the land was the only daughter, who had married and was living in Isahaya. I went to Isahaya and explained my situation to her. She was very kind and generous to let me buy the small lot. She told me, "My father would be glad to know that another doctor is going to stay on his old land."

She sold me the land for a modest price. It was a strange coincidence that a survivor of the atomic bomb would live on the land where an elder graduate of the same medical school lived until he died from the bomb.

When I was trying to find money for the land, a young clerk at the hospital offered to lend me the needed sum of money at no interest. I was surprised by his generosity and accepted his kind offer. We secured the land for our house by good luck and by the good will of this young man. The size of the land was only 153.42 square meters, but it was big enough for our small house. I designed the basic plan of the house and went to the bank to fill out the application form to borrow from the special fund for the private home builder. The chance seemed dim, but I prayed for good luck.

I left Nagasaki with Miwa for Yokohama, where an LST, the American Navy transport ship, was waiting for us *GARIOA* students. Our night in a small inn was miserable. We were victims of bedbugs. But the next morning of July 13 was a beautiful day. Miwa came with me until I boarded the SS Collins which will take me to the United States, but could not stay any longer. It was too hard for her to stand on the shore waving her hand to give a long, hard farewell to me with nobody else to console her. She hurried to the station and took a train to Nagasaki. Her tears did not stop till she got back to Nagasaki, twenty-four hours later.

# PART II

# 10

# A *GARIOA* STUDENT

Our room was on the lowest deck of the ship. It looked like a warehouse with lines of countless hammocks. The ship was built as a navy transport ship to carry as many soldiers as possible in the limited space. One should not expect a nice room. Yet it was much nicer than the ship in which I had been carried to Manchuria. It was much more congenial. Besides, it was no longer wartime. We were allowed up onto the main deck and walked freely and talked with each other after introducing ourselves.

I gazed at the man in front of me when he told me his name was Kagano-Miya, which was the name of a family related to the Emperor. He told me that he had graduated from Tokyo University and was now going to Harvard University. It was my first experience of meeting someone who should be addressed "Miya-sama," a respectful title for certain relatives of the Imperial family. My curiosity was stimulated. He was a nice young gentleman, not much different from an ordinary human being. We did not talk much, but I have remembered this brief encounter all these years.

A voyage on the Pacific Ocean was not as peaceful as the name suggests. By the first evening, the sea became rough. Many passengers became sick by the next morning. I could not eat. I vomited coffee as soon as I drank it. Even the sight of a coffee cup made me nauseated. I could not eat or drink anything. Nausea came up whenever the ship pitched or rolled. Climbing up to the deck, holding a handrail, I tried to breathe the air. But the splash from the high waves would not allow me to stay on deck. I had to rush down and stay in my hammock, feeling nauseous and longing for the end of this miserable voyage.

Good news was announced. The ship would arrive at San Francisco one day earlier than expected. The sea had been rough because the ship took the northern route of the Pacific to navigate faster on the Black Current. Another cause of our seasickness was the small size of the ship.

As we approached the West Coast of America, the sea became quiet and our outlook brighter. I climbed up to the open deck with other passengers and looked to the east, searching for the American continent. At last on July 27, a tip of the continent came into our sight, then it grew larger and larger as we approached San Francisco Bay. The sky was blue without a cloud.

"Look! There is the Golden Gate Bridge!"

Everyone rushed to the eastern side of the deck and watched the familiar shape of the bridge in the distance. A strip of white, shining sand was visible beyond the bridge. It grew to white sky-scrapers and white houses reflecting the summer sunshine. The great city of San Francisco overwhelmed us. Many cars were crossing the Golden Gate Bridge. Soon the Bridge passed over our heads and went behind the ship, which slowly approached the wharf. We were about to take our first steps on the American soil.

Most Americans would not believe that we stayed three days in the dormitory of Mills College, because the college was exclusively for women. We did not know where we were going until our bus stopped at Mills College, Oakland. Neither did we know that the college was a famous women's college. At least I did not. That was why I was shocked when I saw young women in short pants striding and chatting in the dining room of the college. I was convinced finally of the reality of the dormitory being for girls when I was introduced to a bedroom with a bright, colorful wall.

A number of students were staying on campus for various reasons, but no student was playing in the school grounds, because it was the summer vacation. I wondered why this college for women had been selected as our first station in the United States. It was big enough to accommodate four hundred from Japan and one hundred from Okinawa, five hundred students in total. Twenty to thirty percent of our group were female. The location was close to the harbor and to the train station. But one of the reasons must have been to show us this famous college. The beautiful campus and its wide, clean lawn appealed to our eyes, which had become accustomed to watching the rough water of the Pacific Ocean for two weeks. The college was founded in 1852, ninety-nine years before our voyage to America. It was one of two famous old colleges for women in the United States, "Wellesley in the East and Mills in the West." Wellesley was opened in 1875, twenty-three years later than Mills.

Life in the dormitory of Mills College was heavenly. The meals were wonderful for us Japanese, who had experienced hungry post-war days. My favorite dessert was canteloupe filled with ice cream. I had never experienced such a tasty dessert before. I could not believe the fact that it was inexpensive in the United States.

I was also shocked when I could not understand the conversation of girls eating in the dining room. I had passed the difficult examination for GARIOA scholarship and had some confidence in my knowledge of English, but my confidence faded during my first evening at Mills. I am grateful to the dormitory mother who restored my confidence. I had no problem understanding her English when she consoled me. "Your English is much better than our girls' English. It is not your disgrace that you did not understand their conversation. They don't speak proper English, as you do. You should not imitate their English." I appreciated her answer and advice. She was as kind and considerate as the American missionary ladies in Nagasaki who had taught me English.

The train trip from Oakland to New York was rather monotonous. I became aware of the enormous size of the United States. For three days the train ran across the plain most of the time. It stopped occasionally at nondescript stations. One can enjoy a train journey in Japan much more.

The residence of our group in New York was the International House on the campus of Columbia University, along the Hudson River. Near the House I found the grave of General Grant, who had visited Nagasaki once. The surrounding lawn was a beautiful green, and one could see the forest on the New Jersey shore of the Hudson. The Japanese students stretched out on the lawn and enjoyed the freedom of this wide American vista entirely different from the narrow confines of Japanese scenery.

Our orientation course started in one of the buildings on the campus of Columbia University. The main lessons were on American history and American, not British, English. The lectures finished at noon. We spent afternoons in discussion or on trips to various places. Other students from European countries were with us, but we could not fully use the opportunity for communication because of our less fluent English and our tendency to form an isolated Japanese group. Nevertheless, we became friends with each other as we visited museums and factories together and took an excursion boat to the Statue of Liberty. I confess that I was fascinated by the beautiful British English and gentle smile of an older woman scholar from Oslo. On the other hand, students from Germany and France spoke English with strange accents and with national pride, if not racial prejudice, looked down on us Japanese students. We kept our distance from them.

The most charming spot in New York was the Cloisters, a medieval museum. As the name indicates, an old cloister in Europe was moved to a peaceful site at the northern end of Manhattan Island. Collections of medieval paintings, sculptures and tapestries are exhibited in this museum. The building itself has a religious atmosphere, and the whole exhibition represents the religious Middle Ages. When the sun sends colorful lights through the stained window glass onto the stone figure lying on the stone coffin, one forgets the present world and feels the atmosphere of the Middle Ages. The city of New York is out of sight. One can see only the Hudson River and a wooded area from the window. Visitors hesitate to make the sound of steps. It is a serene, sacred place. One can hardly believe that he is in twentieth century New York.

Riverside Church was also on the campus of Columbia University. Famous Reinhold Niebuhr was the preacher. On our first Sunday in New York, I attended this church. I was not impressed as much as I expected. Probably my understanding of his English was insufficient, or perhaps he was better in his writing than in preaching. What impressed me more was the painting hung on a wall of the church. It was the original picture of "Christ Praying in Gethsemane."

After the service, a gentleman approached me. He was a scholar working for the American Geographical Society. He kindly invited me and Mr.Fukuda, who went to the church with me, to his home for lunch. He took us in his car to his house in New Jersey, driving over the George Washington Bridge across the Hudson River. The house was near a large lake in a forest. We appreciated his kindness in inviting us, strangers from Japan. At the entrance of the house, a boy wearing a suit and a necktie hesitantly welcomed us. He was a son of this scholar. He sat quietly listening to our conversation without saying a word unless he was asked. I was impressed by the good manners of this primary school boy. I found that the behaviour of young people depends much upon the family they were brought up by. Children of gentlemen grow up as gentlemen. I learned it in this home of an American geographer.

Not all my impressions of New York were good. My camera was stolen in New York. It happened inside the International House. While I was eating in the dining room, a woman near my seat started to talk about Japan. Since we could not finish our discussion at the dining table, we walked out onto the lawn in front of the grave of General Grant to continue our discussion among the sun-bathing students. After a while I remembered that I had left my camera in the dining room. I jumped up and went back to the table where I was eating. The woman helped me in my search for the lost camera, but we could not find it. I asked waiters and the man at the front table. No one knew about my camera, which was hung on my chair until someone took it and disappeared. I gave up, although it was hard to give up the new Konica camera which I borrowed from a camera shop in Nagasaki, because my friend, the owner of the shop, told me, "You can pay me when you come back from the United States."

It was a brand-new camera. How could I give up? I decided to look for it in all the camera shops of New York. I made a list of them, and started to visit every shop to find the lost camera. It took several days before I realized the uselessness of my desperate search. At the last shop I visited, a man in the shop sympathized with me and recommended a used Kodak camera. He fixed this camera for me and sold it at a reasonable price. It was heavier than the lost Konica, but it was a handy folding camera which could be put into a pocket after folding. I am proud of a masterpiece picture of the Cloisters I photographed with this cheap, old camera.

I am sure the thief was not an American, because the residents of the International House were students from foreign countries. Many of them came from countries struggling to recover from the serious damage of the war. Japan was no exception.

Under U.S. occupation, we were not allowed to carry a single dollar with us. The small amount of money we received on our arrival in New York was scarcely enough to meet our need. I had to wash dishes in the International House to get free meals. I could hardly wait for the day when I could leave New York.

# 11

# ANN ARBOR, MICHIGAN

Ann Arbor is a small town in the suburbs of Detroit. According to Webster's Dictionary published in 1948, the population of Ann Arbor was 29,315. In the fall of 1951, however, there must have been many more in Ann Arbor. A special scholarship was available to young soldiers who had fought in the war, and more than thirty-thousand students were registered in the University of Michigan alone.

My first surprise in Ann Arbor, which I saw from our bus, was a beautiful tunnel of red and yellow leaves over the main street. I had never seen such an avenue decorated with colorful trees in Japan. I felt as if I was welcomed to Ann Arbor by this arch of red, yellow, and orange leaves. What a blissful environment! How lucky I am that I can study in this peaceful town filled with rich trees and wide spaces! I loved the University of Michigan much more than Columbia University, although I missed the view of the Hudson River.

The School of Public Health is located near the University Hospital. It is not a part of the Medical School. It is a postgraduate school where medical doctors or registered nurses study Public Health. It provided no opportunity for clinical experience, but gave the Master's degree in Public Health after one year of study. That is not bad. I should have no complaint because I am studying on a scholarship.

Looking at the program of the public health administration course, I was scared, because medical statistics were among the subjects of study. Neither had I confidence in bacteriology, public health education, maternal and child hygiene, administrative management, and so on.

I was the only Japanese student in the School of Public Health. Other Asian students were a Taiwanese physician, a woman doctor and a male doctor from Thailand. All the others were white except a black doctor in American Army uniform. The nasal intonation and rapid speech of American English were difficult for me to understand. It was easier to talk with students of other nationalities, except an Australian girl. It took me quite a time before I became used to Australian English.

I felt no inferiority complex when I talked with European classmates who spoke slowly with their own accent. It was quite natural to feel close to German students, because we had fought together as allied nations in the last war and were defeated, occupied and prosecuted by foreign forces. We had common experiences and common problems. We understood and sympathized with each other. One of my German classmates was Lilly Wendt, a short blond girl. She wore a happy smile and everyone loved her. She spoke with a strong German accent, which cured my inferiority complex about my English. She was brought up in a well-known family in Germany, but her parents were killed and their estates were taken by the East German Government. She was a health educator in Stuttgart, West Germany. We shared our common experience of the war and common feelings as citizens of defeated nations.

GARIOA students received free tuition and a monthly allowance of 150 dollars. I thought it should be enough for a student, but I was surprised when I was charged 75 dollars a month for my one-room apartment. I had to live on the other half of the allowance. Not much money was left after I sent a sum of money to Miwa. I could not afford to eat every meal in a restaurant. I ate lunch at the inexpensive cafeteria in the school, and the rest of my meals I prepared in my room, which was equipped with a refrigerator and cooking facilities. My routine breakfast was milk and cornflakes. My supper was a unique one consisting of cooked California rice mixed with green peas and ground meat colored with tomato ketchup. I ate it every evening. This simple menu required shopping only once a week, saving my time and money. On Sunday, I ate at a restaurant, often in a Chinese restaurant. This frugal student made a big mistake one Sunday. It was Thanksgiving Day. I went to a church in Ann Arbor. The church was filled with people. The service had started already. I was guided to a front seat. As soon as I sat on the seat, there came a black bag held by a church member in front of my face. When I reached into my purse for an offering, I could not find anything but a five-dollar note. My neighbor was waiting for his turn impatiently. I had no choice. I pulled out the only money I had and put it into the bag. As a new Japanese student in Ann Arbor, I could not disgrace my country by refusing to make an offering. How careless I was, entering a church without coins to offer! This Thanksgiving Day will change to a fasting day for me. I was stupid. I felt miserable. I could not concentrate on the sermon.

When I came out of the church after the service, the minister was waiting for me at the entrance and he spoke to me,"Welcome to our church today. I would like to invite you to our house for dinner. Please, come with me."

I was surprised and then ashamed. He must have thought I listened to his sermon ardently in the front seat, deeply moved by his speech, with my eyes out of focus and my mind in meditation flying out of the world. Actually I was out of my mind at my stupidity in offering all the money I had. What could I have answered if he had asked me about the sermon, to which I was not listening at all? I did not know why he invited me. Was it sympathy for a hungry, new foreign student? Did he intend to treat my homesickness? He might be interested in Japan, because I was the only student who was invited to his home. After all, he noticed me, a poor lonely student sitting in the first row, and kindly invited me as a Thanksgiving Day guest. I had no objection to eating a decent meal. I followed him to his car and to his parsonage.

A little girl of primary school age and her mother welcomed us at the door. The tall, lean pastor tried to relax me with his warm smile and friendly words. Grilled chicken instead of a turkey was served in this pastor's home. It was not a wealthy home, but it was a home of kind hearts and laughter. My empty stomach was filled with satisfaction. I was content. In this kind home of an American pastor, I had no regret that I had paid five dollars for this Thanksgiving Day dinner. I have received his greeting card every Christmas season ever since.

There was a "Campus Chapel" in Ann Arbor. The following Sunday I attended the service at the Campus Chapel. The church belonged to a conservative denomination, but was attended by students and people who work in the university. I felt at home. After the service, coffee was served in a large basement hall. Everyone introduced each other and chatted together. I was treated as an old friend. It was a typical American atmosphere, but I had some difficulty following the American English. It was natural that I approached people who had less American accent. My long friendship started with a Canadian couple named Paul and Mary Jo Miller and a Swiss, Gilbert Beguin, in this Chapel. Paul was studying English literature. His correct, refined English protected my English from the German influence of Lilly Wendt. Mary Jo was an amiable redhead who invited me to their sweet home in a basement.

I more frequently visited the Nunns' home, however. I met this British couple, graduates from the University of London, at a home party on the second day of their arrival in Ann Arbor. G. Raymond Nunn was a scholar of Asian literature. He was able to read Chinese characters, and he spoke Japanese fairly well. During the war he was an information officer in the Indian Division of the British Army and took care of the Japanese prisoners of war. His knowledge of Japan was rich and profound enough to surprise me often. In Ann Arbor he worked in the University Library and studied Chinese and Japanese literature. Sometimes I was useful to him, and he helped me, too. He was a living example of the King's English. His newly married bride Margaret played the piano beautifully, and spoke to me in a delightful English with her wide-opened eyes set on mine without a blink. She had a charming personality.

This newly married couple welcomed me whenever I visited their apartment or "flat," and not only served me British tea but also filled my hungry stomach with British style meals. Once started, we forgot to stop our happy conversation. They were new to America, and did not have many friends. For them my English was more acceptable than American English with its unfamiliar expression and intonation. They had no childen yet, and treated me as a member of their family, although they accepted me even after they had a new baby, calling me "Uncle Martin."

The Roman spelling of my given name is either "Masasiti" or "Masashichi," which is difficult for any foreigner to pronounce and remember. My non-Japanese friends called me Martin. I adopted this Christian name,which was not unfamilar to me, because I was called "Machan" in my childhood. Catholics in Nagasaki have Christian names in addition to their given Japanese names. Martin is a good Christian name. Martin also must be a familiar Christian name in Germany, because there are communities called Martin and the first name of the German reformer was also Martin.

Later in Basel, I found Martin Platz. In the center of this plaza stood a statue of St. Martin, a knight on a horse giving his robe to a man. St. Martinus was born in Hungary in 317. According to legend, he was a Roman soldier with a kind heart. When he saw a naked beggar on a cold street, he cut his robe in two and gave one half to this man, who was Christ himself. He entered a monastery. His final post was Archbishop of Tours, where he served the city well until he died at eighty years of age. He is the Guardian Saint of France. On St. Martin's Day, November 11, a Franciscan sister of St. Francisco Hospital in Nagasaki used to send me a greeting card every year until she died in 1981.

I was scared by the very name of statistics, but fortunately my study of this subject required no advanced mathematics. All calculation was done by an electric counting machine. The computer in 1951 was not so much advanced as it is now. Yet it was good enough to make quick calculations without a mistake, once I learned how to use it. I was amazed at the efficiency of a big IBM machine, which coped with all difficult statistics in a few seconds. All I had to do was to fill the IBM cards and throw them into the machine. No mathematical skill was needed. To my amazement, the report card received evaluating my study of statistics was marked "A." I could not believe it. All credit should go to the IBM machine, which did all the calculations for me. The computer saved me from my inferiority complex in mathematics.

Other subjects were harder than statistics. In an American college, lectures are not the only aspect of education. Students are required to read books on many topics. It was not easy for me to read many pages of many books in English to prepare for the next lecture. Preparation took so much time that I had little time left for anything else. Fortunately the University Library was open until late in the evening on Saturday. Here in this school I had to pass all the tests in one year to get the Master's degree of Public Health.

No extension was possible. I visited the Nunns' home often to enjoy a brief time with them. Once a week I took a piano lesson from a conductor of the choir in the Campus Chapel. But I never studied so hard in Japan as I did in Ann Arbor.

Time passed fast. At the end of the last semester, I had "A"s in nearly all sixteen subjects of my study, except for a few "B"s. I was qualified to receive the Master's degree.

On June 14, 1952, I was graduated from the University of Michigan. The graduation ceremony was called "Commencement." I like this word because it means “beginning". It was not an end. It was a beginning, the start of a new life and a new battle. The final study and hard training begins here. It was a ceremony to encourage new warriors of life.

The place of commencement was not inside a building. It was held in the big football stadium, where exciting football games made people go wild. Led by a brass band in bright uniforms, new graduates wearing dark gowns and square caps proceeded onto the ground. I was one of them. I saw Ray and Margaret smiling in the stands. The President of the University spoke first, followed by the speeches of distinguished guests. At the end, the names of the graduates were called one after another, and diplomas were handed out. My turn came and I stood in front of the President. I sent a smile to the Nunns. They returned my smile. I shouted in my heart, "I owe you this honor. I thank you."

The Commencement came to an end. All the graduates shouted aloud with joy and happiness, and ran to their families and relatives to embrace each other. I had no family or relative, but Ray and Margaret Nunn hurried to congratulate me. The Millers were also present, and congratulated me on my graduation. I knew Miwa was also congratulating me in Nagasaki.

# 12

# GLEN LAKE, MINNESOTA

It was a long bus ride. Leaving Ann Arbor in the afternoon, the Greyhound bus passed Chicago at midnight. On the next morning the bus was running through the vast plain of Wisconsin. No mountain was visible. Wild land and cultivated field appeared in turn. A river came into view. I was told that it was the Mississippi River. I was surprised to find the Mississippi in this North-Central region. I knew the river flowed into the Gulf of Mexico after flowing through the southern states but I did not know that it started in Minnesota, a northern state. Even in the state of Minnesota, this great, slowly flowing river looked wider than Japanese rivers.

Bridges welcomed us one after another as our bus approached the city of St. Paul. The next city across the river was Minneapolis. As the name of the Twin Cities may suggest, the two cities are separated by the Mississippi River. Minneapolis is larger and has taller buildings. A passenger told me that the highest building I saw in Minneapolis was the Forshey Tower, The Greyhound stopped at the bus terminal in Minneapolis at last, but this terminal was not my destination. I had to take another bus going to "Oak Terrace." The bus went through the city of Minneapolis, ran along a beautiful lake, passed a small town, and then came to the open suburbs. Driving around the forest of white birches shining in the evening sun, the bus finally stopped in front of a large building. It was the Glen Lake Sanatorium.

The University of Michigan granted me the Master's degree, but provided no clinical experience. My ambition to learn the technique of lung resection was not satisfied. From Ann Arbor I had written a letter to Rev. Ernie Best in Nagasaki. Rev. Best came to Nagasaki as a missionary from Canada after the war. He bought some burnt land in Shiroyama, near Takeno-kubo, and built a small

"Peace Memorial Church." I was asked to correct the Japanese manuscripts of his Sunday sermon. Every other Sunday I substituted for him at the service until I left Nagasaki, because speaking in Japanese was not easy for this Canadian missionary. Shortly before Commencement, I received his letter telling me that he had arranged for me to work at the State Sanatorium in Glen Lake as a resident. The Director of the Sanatorium was his old friend. I was thankful to Providence for offering me such a good opportunity.

A tall, gray-haired physician welcomed me at the Director's Office. He joked, "Best is my best friend," and called Dr. Victor Funk, who was to take care of me. Dr. Funk appeared. He was a man of medium size and a powerful build. He smiled at me and gripped my hand with his thick, strong hand. I was also introduced to his colleague, Dr. Frances King. She was not a king but a queen with a stately figure and a gentle smile.She had been a missionary doctor in China before she came home. She welcomed me as another Asian doctor. There were already two other Asian doctors from China.

This State Sanatorium had more than 500 beds, but the number of the staff was less than ten, fewer than at Ureshino Hospital. Dr. Funk and I had to take care of fifty patients, too many to remember each name. Yet Dr. Funk called every patient by name during his morning round. I was amazed at his good memory. It might not be amazing, because TB patients stay long in the same hospital. I too made the effort to remember their names. I was delighted to find a Japanese name among my patients. She was Kuwa Yoshida, a Nisei Japanese. She spoke Japanese with some difficulty. She preferred to talk to me in English. She helped me in many ways.

As I expected, pulmonary surgery was performed frequently every week.The chief operator was Dr. Thomas Kinsella, a chest surgeon from the University of Minnesota. Dr. Funk and I assisted him. The instrument nurse was Miss Mary Shonka. She handed the right surgical instrument to the surgeon at the right moment without wasting time. She knew all the procedures and the choice of instruments. Her sharp sense and quick movement impressed me. But if I made any mistake or acted too slowly, her big, blue, scorching eyes stared at me. I was scared.

Pneumonectomy is a technique to cut off the infected lung lesion with the tuberculous cavity. But total removal of one lung was seldom done. Partial resection of the lung was more common. It was not easy to separate the upper lobe from the middle or the lower lobes because of adhesion to each other and to the thoracic wall. If the thin membrane covering the lung is damaged, the air leaks from the lung and the remaining lung loses its function. Attempts to repair the torn membranes often enlarge the damage. Indeed poor repair work to the damaged lung often caused the failure of early pneumonectomy. In Glen Lake Sanatorium the surgeon used a special gastrectomy clamp to cut the lung. The border between the normal and diseased areas of the lung was clipped with this long clamp and the diseased portion was resected. The clamp was removed after air-tight suturing of the end line as in the case of gastric resection. No leakage of air or bleeding from the cut end resulted from this technique. Its advantage is that a surgeon can remove only the diseased lesion of the lung, without sacrificing the entire lobe or lung. Following this kind of surgery, the function of the remaining lung was much better than one could anticipate with earlier surgical techniques.

There was a patient called Ida Myring whose one lung was totally damaged by tuberculosis bacilli. Her vital capacity was only 900 cc, one third of the normal average for women. She panted often after every movement. She was scheduled for total pneumonectomy of her left lung, because her right lung was intact. She was a small, lovely housewife who had a friendly smile for everyone. I was not sure if she could stand the long major surgery to remove one lung entirely, but she did not show any anxiety before the surgery. My worry was unnecessary. The surgery was successful. When she woke up from anesthesia, she smiled at us and thanked us. I did not believe that she would live long, but she went home while I was in Glen Lake. Thirty-two years later, in 1984, I visited her at her home in Minneapolis. She welcomed me with her nice familiar smile. Though over seventy years of age, she was doing her household work like other housewives. Her vital capacity had increased to 1200 cc. I was glad for her. She survived so many years because she had had tuberculosis instead of fatal cancer of the lung.

As the name of Glen Lake suggests, there was a lake called Glen Lake near the sanatorium. It was a small lake. Ten minutes' ride from the sanatorium there was a larger, well-known lake called Lake Minnetonka. "Minne" means water in an Indian language. "Minneapolis" means a city of water. The State of Minnesota is a state of many lakes. It was no wonder that this state, filled with lakes and silver birches, attracted immigrants from Scandinavian countries, from Norway and Sweden in particular. That was why there were many "Larsons" and "Petersons" among the nurses in Glen Lake Sanatorium. When I forgot the name of a nurse, I called her "Miss Larson." One of the doctors was also Dr. Larson, a typical Norwegian, tall with blond hair. Nearly all the patients had blond hair, for they were also Norwegians. My black hair was a disharmony in Glen Lake. When I was sitting with nurses at a table one evening, one of them surprised me, saying, "The nurses admire your jet black hair."

We Asians envy the blond hair of Westerners. It had never occurred to me that people with blond or brown hair could envy our black hair. I did not know then that there is a song, "Black is the color of my true love's hair." My inferiority complex owing to the disagreeable color of my hair disappeared completely in this hospital, thanks to a nurse's complimenting words about my hair. Nor did I mind my flat nose any more, since I learned that many Western women dislike their high-sticking noses. It is foolish for Japanese women to dye their hair blond or brown and to elevate their nose by plastic surgery. It is also foolish for white or oriental women to curl their long, straight hair, while there are black women who try to make their hair straight. We should be more natural, keeping our own heritages.

Only one Japanese patient stayed in Glen Lake Sanatorium, but Kuwa told me that there were many Japanese living in Minneapolis. On Sunday her parents took me to the Twin City Independent Church between St. Paul and Minneapolis. The church was for Japanese Americans. They had no chapel of their own. They used a hall in the YMCA for Sunday services.

There was a missionary lady named Miss Evans, who had been the principal of a mission school in Sapporo, Japan until she retired. This sweet old lady was living in Minneapolis with her sister, and played the organ on Sunday at the service. The pastor was a Nisei Japanese. He preached to the Nisei audience in English, but he had difficulty in preaching to older Japanese in Japanese. As soon as he heard about my background, he asked me to preach on Sunday to the Issei Japanese. I felt my obligation to speak on the Gospel for those old Japanese Americans who immigrated to the United States before the war and were driven from the West Coast to the Midwest camps to live in confinement and suffering until the end of the war, then had to start again in the Midwest where their children found jobs. Every Sunday I attended the Japanese church faithfully from that day, and found new Christian friends among them.

Minnesota is heavenly in the autumn. Surrounding the lakes there are many woods and forests. Green leaves of trees change to red, brown, orange and yellow colors in the whole state. As soon as one leaves the Twin Cities, woods, lakes, and forests form a beautiful panorama of this blessed land. One can enjoy the endless, blue sky and unspoiled nature. One seldom sees houses. One day a young couple took me to an Indian village. I was overwhelmed by the grandeur of nature embracing the village. That night feather-headed Indians danced around a big communal fire under the full moon.

The autumn was, however, too short. The first snow came in October. The leaves suddenly disappeared from the trees, and no evergreens were visible. The temperature went down day by day. One could not walk outdoors without a heavy overcoat. The temperature of -45°C is equivalent to the winter temperature at the northern end of Hokkaido in northern Japan. In this central region of the North American continent, the difference in temperature between day and night is bigger than at the coast. The November snow stayed without melting. The nurses' dormitory was connected to the sanatorium by an underground tunnel. Transportation was a big problem. Surgery was often cancelled when the anesthesiologist could not get to the hospital. It was the longest winter I have ever experienced in my life.

Fortunately I was a resident. I occupied a large room in the basement, and I was on duty every night. One night I woke up to a sudden, blinding light. I found a night supervisor nurse looking at my bed with a flashlight in her hand. She explained that she came down because I had not answered her telephone call. Usually I responded well to a telephone call. Often in the evening Kuwa called me. I was needed as a bridge game member. Other members of the team were a tall gentleman with a mustache and an elderly spinster. They taught me how to play bridge. Occasionally glancing at the snowfall through the frozen window we enjoyed this pastime on long winter nights.

When the Christmas season came, there were many happy events, including a Christmas pageant and a Christmas concert. I was invited to the Children's Ward on Christmas night. I enjoyed singing Christmas songs with the children, and listened to the harp played by a nurse named Miss Louise Knoki. The peaceful sound of the harp was fascinating. It was a wonderful Christmas.

Spring came suddenly to Minnesota. In mid-April, the snow started to melt. The air became softer and tempted us outdoors. All around the sanatorium, yellow flowers filled the earth. Later feathers of dandelions fly up to the sky. Willow trees sprout thin leaves. The green leaves of silver birches rattle in the wind. "Spring has come, spring has come," everyone wants to sing the song of the spring. Butterflies and bees thronged to Glen Lake, and the patients went out into the open yard. Tables and chairs were brought out and outdoor parties were filled with joyful voices. I joined them often. I was also invited to a picnic on the lake. I felt that I had belonged to Glen Lake Sanatorium for years.

Summer returned again to Glen Lake. It meant my departure. I left Glen Lake after saying farewell to my dear patients, nurses and doctors. At Minneapolis Airport, nearly all the Twin City Japanese Church members came to see me off. When I came to Minnesota one year earlier, I had no friends here. After living one year in Minnesota, I had the privilege of knowing many nice people. I will miss them. I thanked God for my experience in Glen Lake Sanatorium.

# 13

# THE SECOND DEPARTMENT OF SURGERY

A new house was waiting for me in Nagasaki. It was a small, sweet home which I had planned before I left Japan and Miwa had built during my stay in the United States. She borrowed money from the Government and hired carpenters and made the house ready for my homecoming. For two full years she waited for me in Nagasaki, earning money by teaching dressmaking at Yuaikan, a settlement house set up by Rev. Best. I did not know how to thank her. From the house I could see Mount Inasa beyond the small garden Miwa had designed. The house faced south and good sunshine filled the house on sunny days. The location of No. 90 Takeno-kubo was not far from Nagasaki Hospital, just the right distance.

Most of my patients had been discharged during the two years of my absence, but the staff were the same. A new doctor, Dr. Hayashi, and a new pharmacist, Mr. Hanada, had been added. The nursing staff did not change much. They were happy to have me again in the hospital.

There were, however, many obstacles to practising my newly acquired surgical technique in this hospital. It was a small hospital originally built for epidemic diseases. It had no surgical setup. There was no surgeon on the staff of five internists and a Medical Director. Thoracoplasty can be performed under local anesthesia, but pneumonectomy requires general anesthesia using endotracheal intubation to send the anesthetic gas and oxygen to the lung and to keep controlled respiration during the surgical exposure of the lung to atmospheric pressure. Pneumonectomy is impossible without an anesthetist and machines for general anesthesia. The

Nagasaki Hospital had none of them. Even in the Medical School Hospital there was no anesthetist at that time.

It was from the Second Department of Surgery, Nagasaki Medical School that I received an invitation to teach surgery. Rebirth of the Nagasaki Medical School was going on in Urakami. The destroyed buildings were repaired and all the clinical departments were moved to Urakami from the Isahaya Hospital in 1951. The Isahaya Hospital was renamed the Isahaya Health Insurance Hospital. The buildings of the Shinkozen Clinic were returned to the former owner, Shinkozen Primary School. Professor Koyano was called back from the Ureshino Hospital to become the Dean of the Medical School again in November, 1952.

The Chief of the Second Department of Surgery was Professor Hideo Tsujimura, and the Associate Professor was Dr. Takashi Hirai, an expert in abdominal surgery. I did not know who proposed my appointment as a lecturer in pulmonary surgery when I came back from the United States, but on the first of February 1954, I was officially appointed as a lecturer in surgery in the medical school.

In the Second Department of Surgery, there were two surgeons who had graduated from the medical school one year earlier than I had. They stayed in the medical school after graduation, as interns at first, then as residents. After more than five years of residency they became paid instructors of surgery. Now I was appointed as a paid lecturer without long residency in the department. It was an unprecedented appointment. It was regarded by the other residents as an intrusion of an outsider. Some of them were angry at the appointment, but they could not complain because there was no one in the department who was capable of performing pneumonectomy. I was needed in the department, but I felt uncomfortable.

The problem of anesthesia had to be solved first. I studied books on anesthesia, remembering what anesthetists were doing at Glen Lake. To practise anesthesia myself, I went to the National Tuberculosis Sanatorium in Kiyose, Tokyo. Their chief surgeon was Dr. Shinobu Miyamoto, who was another GARIOA student. There was also Dr. Ryohei Koga, who was once an intern in Ureshino Hospital, as I had been. They provided me with the opportunity to see and practise anesthesia. The anesthetist was Dr.T.

Morioka, who later became Professor of Anesthesiology in Kumamoto University. I learned all the techniques of general anesthesia and mastered the difficult endotracheal intubation before I came back to Nagasaki.

Fortunately there was a young doctor who had an interest in anesthesiology in the Second Department of Surgery. He was Dr. Yutaka Goto, who later became Professor of Anesthesiology at Nagasaki University. He soon developed his skill in anesthesia, and became a good anesthetist before long. He was dependable. I let him work on anesthesia while I concentrated on surgery of the lung. With his good cooperation, I operated on many tuberculous lungs in the following years. Most of the surgeries were partial resections. I removed the diseased part of the lung as I learned at Glen Lake. All went well. We had no postoperative infection thanks to chemotherapy developed in Japan after the war. Our good result attracted many cases of pulmonary tuberculosis to our Department. Other residents who assisted me gradually mastered the technique of pneumonectomy. Some of them operated by themselves without my help.

My surgical experience in pneumonectomy had reached nearly one hundred cases when I encountered a case of extensive chronic infection of the lung filled with pus. The patient was a young woman, one of whose lungs had lost its function. We decided to remove the whole lung because the other lung was intact. The operation took a long time, because the lung was adhered to the chest wall tightly by repeated infection. Carefully we freed the lung from the thoracic wall and disconnected the bronchus and blood vessels before we took out the lung. We closed the large wound with tight sutures, leaving a drainage tube in the thorax, and came out of the operating room for a rest.

Before long I was notified that something was wrong with the patient. I ran to her. She was already in a state of shock. Her face was pale, her pulse was weak, and her blood pressure was critically low. A blood transfusion was given, and injection of drugs was repeated, but her condition did not improve. I decided to open the chest again to look inside the thorax. It was filled with blood. Blood was leaking from the cut end of an artery which had been tied once but must have become loose. Perhaps the tie was not tight enough. But whatever the immediate cause of this mishap, it is the surgeon who must finally be blamed. I tried everything to save her life, but the situation was hopeless. She died eventually. Her dead face was so beautiful that I could not hold back my tears.

Recovery from my grief was not easy. I was discouraged too much by the first post-operative death of my patient. I lost my enthusiasm for lung surgery. By that time I had trained several surgeons for lung surgery in the department. They were good enough to operate on the lung. I was no longer needed. What should I do next?

The next target of chest surgery should be the heart. But cardiac surgery needs a team of doctors. It cannot be done single-handed as in lung surgery, and I had little hope of getting enough staff to help me do heart surgery in my department. Besides, the First Department of Surgery had already started on a heart surgery project, led by ProfessorTsuji himself. One department is enough for heart surgery in one university. I should look for some other field of surgery in which no one in our school was engaged.

While I was pondering what I should study next, an unforgettable incident took place. A veteran surgeon was operating on a case of brain tumor. I was watching his operation because I had had no experience in brain surgery. The surgery was a failure. From the beginning of this craniotomy there was uncontrollable bleeding of the brain. The surgeon tried to stop the bleeding, but he could not control it. He gave up and put the bone flap back over the bleeding brain and closed the scalp in a hurry. The tumor was untouched. The blood-stained surgeon looked at me and said in a cynical way,"This is not unusual in surgery of the brain." I shouted in my mind, "It should not be that way."

Brain surgery had been done in the past in our Medical School Hospital. But the cases were few. Most craniotomies were done to treat head injuries. There were a few reports of successful removal of parasites from the brain, but the successful removal of a brain tumor was not reported. Surgeons were not interested in brain surgery. No one had wanted to be a neurosurgeon in Nagasaki Medical School so far. Somebody must fill the gap. If no one else intended to study neurosurgery, I should do it. I made up my mind.

The history of neurosurgery is rather new. It is true that many operated skulls were found in Peru, suggesting that surgical operations had been performed in Ancient Peru, and trephination was attempted in the Greco-Roman world and in medieval times, too. But it was at the end of the last century when the first surgeon specializing in neurosurgery appeared in history. He was Sir Victor Horsley (1857-1916) of England. Rapid progress in this century owes much to Dr. Harvey Cushing, a pioneer neurosurgeon in America. He died in 1939, but his followers brought to America a golden age of neurosurgery. Progress in Japan was slower. Only a few pioneers, including Dr. Mizuho Nakata, Professor of Niigata University, Dr. Kentaro Shimizu, Professor of Tokyo University, and Dr. Senri Araki, Professor of Kyoto University, studied neurosurgery in the United States and trained their disciples in neurosurgery before the War. It was only in post-war Japan that neurosurgery was studied by many Japanese surgeons. In Kyushu University, Associate Professor Dr. Jinnai was trying to develop neurosurgery in Kyushu.

As soon as I had made a plan to visit Niigata University where Professor Nakata was teaching neurosurgery, I flew to Niigata. Professor Nakata introduced me to his Associate Professor Ueki, who kindly made arrangements for my stay and my observation of brain surgery. He answered all my basic questions with patience. One week spent in Niigata was a good introduction to clinical neurosurgery, even though it was far too short to gain a basic knowledge of neurosurgery. It was enough, however, to set my mind on the study of neurosurgery.

I wrote a letter to Dr. Takao Mitsuno, Professor of Surgery, Iwate Medical School, asking him to introduce me to a good institute in the United States to study neurosurgery. He had been my senior member of Saga High School Bible Study Group. After graduation from Kyushu University, he studied neurosurgery and wrote a good textbook on neurosurgery. He became famous for his successful surgeries on intracranial hypertensive hemorrhage.

He recommended me to Professor George Austin of the University of Oregon Medical School. He was a friend of Dr. Austin, who had studied neurosurgery under Professor Fraser in the University of Pennsylvania and was Associate Professor until he was invited by the University of Oregon as a new Professor of Neurosurgery. He needed new residents and asked Professor Mitsuno to recommend Japanese residents. Two Japanese surgeons were recommended, but Dr. George Austin preferred me to another surgeon from Iwate, because I had already had experience of residency in the United States and had less difficulty in English. I appreciated the kind recommendation of Professor Mitsuno.

I had no difficulty obtaining permission from Nagasaki Medical School to study abroad. Although it was my second opportunity to study in the United States, it was my first overseas study since I came to the Second Department of Surgery four years earlier. My basic salary would be paid for two years, enough to guarantee the needs of Miwa who must stay at home, but I did not have enough money for my flight to Portland,Oregon. I wrote a letter to Dr. Austin, asking him to lend me money for a flight ticket from Japan to Portland. He sent me a ticket by return mail. I promised him to repay the expense from my allowance in Oregon. The allowance would not be much, but I would be able to repay him within one or two years in his Department of Neurosurgery because a room and meals were provided for a resident.

I have an old photograph which was taken in January, 1958 in front of the Imperial Palace. There is a boy between Miwa and me. He was Toshio,who had lived with us for three years already and was adopted as our son by this time. He came to Tokyo with Miwa to see me off. Miwa would not cry this time in the train on her way back to Nagasaki, because she was not alone. This time she did not have to stand on the pier of Yokohama holding a long ribbon and waving her hand for a long time, because my plane took off from Haneda Airport within a few minutes. The day was January 6, two days after my fortieth birthday.

# 14

# A NEUROSURGICAL RESIDENT IN PORTLAND, OREGON

The airplane arrived at Portland, Oregon, before dawn. The sky was dark until I came up to the entrance of the Medical School Hospital of the University of Oregon, after passing through the sleeping city of Portland and up the hill leading to the hospital. I walked into the lobby to the front desk and told a woman who I was. She was expecting me and guided me to a resident room on the fourth floor. I placed my luggage on the floor and approached the window. The cloudy sky had a scarlet color. The crossing lines of streets under the cloud were still dim, but all the streets were clearly outlined by street lights. On the dark streets were running headlights and taillights like a moving chain of jewels. Far beyond the streets there was a river with the forests and sky in the background, a beautiful view. As I watched, the sky changed its color to orange and a silhouette of a mountain similar to Mt. Fuji rose up from the horizon. What a happy surprise to see the image of Mt.Fuji in this remote land of Oregon! The name of the mountain was St. Helens, I was told later.

"Welcome, Dr. Kawano." Professor George Austin smiled at me and shook my hand. He was a handsome gentleman of medium size and healthy figure. He must have been in his early forties, but his brownish blond hair was mixed with gray. He was a mountaineer, with ready-to-be-released reserves of energy behind his gentle smile. He looked unpredictable. There were two windows in his office and the sun was illuminating a heap of writing papers on his desk. A gray-haired secretary saluted me with a smile. I expected a cup of tea or coffee to come from her corner. But Professor Austin was not waiting for tea. He announced: "Now, shall we go to the wards to make a round visit?" I was not ready, because I expected a different remark, such as, "You must be tired after a long trip. You may rest all day today."

I gave him my consent, however, and followed him to the wards, because I thought he wanted to introduce me to the patients and nurses in the neurosurgical wards. As soon as we reached the eighth floor, the round visit started. Without introducing me to the head nurse who followed us, he visited every patient in the wards, giving me a comment on each patient. No other doctor came with us. When the morning round finished, he ordered me, "Wash your hands to be ready for surgery. We'll start surgery now."

I followed him to the surgical theater. No one else was scrubbing. The two of us washed our hands, sterilized them and went into the operating room. I found no other surgeon in the room, but an ananesthetist and a nurse. I thought we were going to operate on a simple case, because only two of us were needed. It was not a simple case, however. It was a craniotomy to remove a brain tumor after sawing out a large bone flap of the skull. It was after noon by the time the operation was finished.

Still I could not find time for rest. After eating a late lunch in the cafeteria, I found a number of examinations waiting for me. There were many radiographic examinations of the brain besides plain skull x- ray films. Angiography demonstrates blood vessels in the brain by injection of a radio-opaque dye into the common carotid artery. The spinal cord is examined by injecting the dye into the spinal lumen through the lumbar spine. Pneumoencephalography is injection of air into cerebral ventricles through a trephine hole of the skull to demonstrate the silhouette of the ventricular system. Dr. Austin demonstrated the former two methods that afternoon. They were not easy tests. When all procedures were finished, he told me,

"You can do these tests by yourself from now on." I was aghast. He added another punch, "We'll start the evening round at 8:30." Then he left the hospital to eat dinner at home.

I ate supper at the cafeteria in the hospital and went to the wards before Dr. Austin came. After the evening round, I had to change the dressing of the operated patient. It was late at night when I reached my room on the fourth floor. My roommate was an intern called Nicolson. After introducing ourselves, he told me about the neurosurgical department in this University of Oregon Medical School Hospital. No other neurosurgeon was in the department, neither assistant nor instructor. The only other resident, who came from France, was ready to leave Oregon and move to the East Coast.

"I can't believe that there is no one but a professor in a department of neurosurgery of a medical school. What happened?"

"In the University of Oregon, there was a skillful neurosurgeon named Dr. Raph. All neurosurgeons practicing in Portland were trained by him. When the University appointed Dr. Austin, a famous scholar from the East, as the Chief of Staff, Dr.Raph resented it and left the University to become the Chief Neurosurgeon at the Good Samaritan Hospital in Portland. All the residents followed him and none of the staff stayed in the University."

Now I understood why Dr. Austin asked Professor Mitsuno, a foreign friend, to recommend Japanese residents. I thought I was lucky, but actually I was caught in a trap. No one in Portland wanted to be his resident. Even the one from France had not wanted to stay. Then I volunteered to work as a resident responsible for all residents' work in this department of neurosurgery, like "a summer fly jumping into the burning fire," as the Japanese say.

There was no returning for me, however. I owed Professor Austin the cost of the long flight from Japan to Portland and had no money for another flight to Japan. As a Japanese who was taught, "Once a man leaves his home for study, he should never come home until he achieves his goal," I should be ashamed to leave this difficult post. As a matter of fact, I had no way to go home. All roads were closed to me. I had no other choice but to stay. I made up my mind to work for one year at least, however hard my work would be, because I came there to study neurosurgery.

It was a busy, hard life, much more than I expected. I had to get up by 6:30, because the morning round started at 7:15. Often I ran to the wards without breakfast. Once or twice I was not on time, and Professor Austin stared at me with scorching eyes.

Surgery started at eight or earlier. This refers to the time for cutting the scalp with a scalpel. To be ready for this moment I had to go to the surgical theater earlier to sterilize my hands and put on a surgical gown and gloves. If I was late, the anesthetist would become nasty. One cannot operate smoothly if he quarrels with the anesthetist. Anesthesiology is a specialized profession. The anesthetist has his own pride, and would not yield to the pressure of a surgeon. I heard a story that Dr. Austin once quarrelled with an anesthetist, and took him to the corridor to settle the matter with his fists. So far in Oregon, he had not fought with anesthetists.

I did not expect so many operations in one department of neurosurgery. There were not only cases of brain surgery but also many cases of spinal cord surgery. The surgery of herniated intervertebral disc was performed frequently by neurosurgeons in the United States. The intervertebral disc between the vertebrae is a kind of cushion to allow flexibility of the spine. If this disc slips out, it will compress the nerves of the spinal cord and cause pain in the hip and legs. Surgical removal of the herniated disc can relieve the pain. This surgery of the disc is done by orthopedic surgeons in Japan for the reason that it is surgery of the bone. But in the United States it is performed by neurosurgeons because it is surgery related to the spinal cord. Dr. Cloward at the University of Hawaii is famous for his approach to the cervical disc through the mouth. He is not an orthopedist but a neurosurgeon. I was embarrassed when he asked me in Honolulu during a cervical disc operation in which I assisted him, "Why do Japanese neurosurgeons let orthopedists do this operation?"

Chordotomy was another common surgery of the spine, second only to disc surgery. "Chord" means the spinal cord. Chordotomy is an operation to cut the spinal cord, not entirely, but only the neural tract conveying the pain sensation. The lateral spinothalamic tract runs along the anterolateral side of the spinal cord towards the brain. The width is only 4.5mm. Along the course of the sensory tract the motor tract runs downwards to mediate orders of the brain to the muscles of the body. If the knife slips and cuts this tract, the lower half of the body will be paralyzed. Chordotomy is a delicate surgery. No overcutting or undercutting is allowed on each side of the spinal cord. How did I know that I would have the fate of performing this chordotomy on my own niece ten years later?

It was not easy to remove the spinal process and vertebrae imbedded in the thick layers of muscles. More difficult still was to control bleeding from the muscles. Dr. Austin demonstrated to me how to operate on the spine speedily with minimum bleeding. It did not take a month before he trusted my skill and let me do the procedure without his help except the vital maneuver. He told me again and again, "You have had experience in surgery for many years. You should be able to do this surgery without my help, if I demonstrate it only once. Remember, you are now our chief resident."

One after another he entrusted me with different neurological procedures, after demonstrating his method. He wanted to save his time for experiments in his laboratory. He was more interested in research and experiment than in surgery. He called me chief resident, but I had to do everything as the only resident in the department. It was too much. I was too busy. I resented the situation. I did not need the honor of being the chief resident. I needed other residents to help me and substitute for me. On the other hand, it was a great opportunity for me to learn all aspects of and procedures in neurosurgery. In a short period I developed my skill in neurological surgery, often working as the chief operator.

There were many cases of brain tumor. I operated on the malignant as well as benign brain tumors. I was amazed to find many brain and spinal cord tumors among children and infants. I loved these children. When one of my children died after long and difficult surgery, I cried with the mother. Then it was my sad duty to ask the mother for permission to autopsy her dead child. Tears came again when the mother replied, "I refuse to let my child be autopsied by any one but you, dear doctor. If you do the autopsy, I will give permission, because you loved her and she loved you."

Patients with pituitary adenoma presented unique pictures. Typical features of acromegaly were the long chin,big nose and enlarged fingertips. Dysfunction of the pituitary gland caused both overgrowth and suspension of growth, giants and pygmies. Visual defects and disorder of the menses were also symptoms of pituitary tumors. Removal of the tumor was not easy, because the pituitary body is located in the base of the brain behind the eyes. Fortunately I experienced no postoperative death, but there was one sad case in pituitary surgery.

A woman with metastatic breast cancer was referred us for pituitary body resection, because the removal of the pituitary body was believed to be effective in preventing metastasis of the cancer. The surgery was successful, but metastases spread. Metastatic cancer of the lung caused pleural fluid and difficulty in breathing. It was painful to see the patient making an effort to breathe, but she joked whenever I approached her and she smiled at me as if she were telling me, "I know what is wrong. I am ready for the worst. Never mind."

Dr. Austin ordered me to do a tracheotomy, but I hesitated. Respiration through the endotracheal tube inserted into the incised trachea would certainly make her breathing easier, but she would not be able to speak a word any more, even when she wanted to say something before dying; too depressing for a conscious patient. It would only be a remedy for a comatose patient who needs more airflow into the lung. I disobeyed Dr. Austin, but he insisted that I do this tracheotomy. I felt miserable as I cut her throat to insert the air tube. She did not refuse me. She nodded to me, looking at my eyes. She understood my situation. I was unhappy even after the surgery. I tried not to see the air tube in her throat, but I had to come to her bed. Every time I visited her she welcomed me with a smile as if to say "I understand you. Don't worry." Our silent conversation did not last long. She expired before long.

Every day there was surgery in the three hospitals, the University Hospital, the County Hospital on the other side of the street, and the Veterans Hospital a few blocks away. In one single day, I had to operate on six cases in twenty-two hours from early morning till late at night. A resident means a doctor living in a hospital. He is on duty every night. I was often called at midnight to treat patients injured in automobile accidents. All cases of head injury and cerebral hemorrhage were my responsibility. I had to operate with an intern. Dr. Austin would not let me rest after my all-night hard labor tackling emergency cases. The next case of surgery was waiting in the morning. I became a victim of chronic headache and indigestion. I felt fever and dizziness sometimes, but Dr. Austin did not pay attention. He said, "Keep working. It will go away." He could not do without me, because there was no other resident in his department.

The shunting operation was a common surgical procedure for hydrocephalus. An obstructed ventricular passway causes dilatation of the ventricles and compression of the brain, leading to death. To relieve the pressure, anastomosis is built with a small by-pass tube between the ventricle and the carotid vein or the abdominal cavity. Eventually this procedure became my responsibility

The stereotactic surgery for Parkinsonism, however, was Dr. Austin's monopoly. It was a complicated procedure to coagulate a certain spot in the mid-brain as a treatment of Parkinsonian tremor. Using an apparatus he had designed, the tip of an electric needle was accurately placed at a certain spot after radiographic test and measurement. It was boring for me, who had not much to do during the long procedure.

The most difficult surgery was that of cerebral aneurysm. Aneurysms in the Willis circle of cerebral arteries are located deep in the base of the skull. The operative field was visible only to the main operator, Dr. Austin. In advance, I had to expose the common carotid arteries and vertebral arteries on both sides and pass rubber bands around the artery to be ready to bind them temporarily when sudden, unexpected bleeding started from the ruptured aneurysm by accidental mismanipulation. It took one whole day to perform aneurysm surgery. Not all aneurysm surgery was successful until microsurgery was introduced by Dr. M. G. Yasargil at the Kantonspital Zurich in the next decade.

Surgery was not all of my work. I had to do angiographic studies of brain arteries on five or six patients a day, in addition to encephalographic study of the ventricle and myelography of the spinal cord. Negotiation with surgical nurses for the use of the surgical theater and with the x-ray department for the arrangement of schedules was also my hazardous duty. I argued with the chief surgical nurse at every emergency operation. Sometimes I wanted to quit. I thought I had had enough. The first two months were the worst period, in which 87 cases were operated, with no other resident to help me. It is unbelievable that I was able to survive the nightmare.

# 15

# EASTER SUNDAY

It was on the morning of Easter Sunday when I met Miss Margaret E. Hughes for the first time. I went to the garden of the Medical School campus on the first Sunday of April 6, because I saw a poster on a board that a morning service would be held in the garden on Easter Sunday. It was a beautiful morning which reminded me of the view I saw on the day of my first arrival at Portland. But the number of people gathered was not many. We sang Easter hymns looking at the dawning sky, and a pastor gave us a brief message of Easter. The service ended sooner than I expected. Then Miss Hughes asked me,

"Would you come with us to have breakfast at my apartment?" "Thank you, Miss Hughes. I would be glad to." Miss Hughes was the Superintendent of the Medical Library. "Please call me Margaret, for I will call you Martin."

Her apartment was only a five minute walk from the hospital. It was not a cold, concrete building, as most Japanese apartments were. It was a long two-story wooden building, and Margaret lived on the first floor. Her apartment was a comfortable set of two rooms and a dining kitchen. In the kitchen there was a small dining table near the window through which one could see nothing but the sky and forest. I felt as if I sat in a bungalow, far from the town. No other house was visible because the building was located at the end of the hill on which the Medical School Hospital stood. I was attracted by this quiet apartment and its peaceful view.

Other guests at the table were a friend of Margaret called Marie and a Filipino student called Makiso. Bread, bacon and fried egg were served. This simple breakfast tasted much more delicious in this room than the breakfast in the hospital cafeteria. Margaret spoke fast, but I understood her English, because she was born in

Canada and brought up in Canada speaking Canadian English. To my surprise, she had worked at the Glen Lake Sanatorium until she moved to Oregon. It was more than a coincidence. I felt as if I met a person who had come from my home town.

After this Easter Sunday, I regularly attended the Sunday service at St. Stephen's Church to which Margaret belonged. It was an Episcopal church, and it took me some time before I became used to the ceremonial service of the church. However, the classic English of the prayer book was beautiful. I enjoyed reading it with the congregation every Sunday.

Margaret asked me to join the church choir. I found out why as soon as I joined the choir. There were four or five bass singers, but only one tenor besides me. The tenor was a semi-professional singer with a good voice, who could accurately read the musical score. I admired his singing and wanted to learn from him. I kept singing in the choir. The score of the new song for each Sunday was handed to us one hour before the service. I could not sing well from the score at the beginning. I tried to follow the fine tenor who sang any new song without an error. I was shocked one Sunday when I could not find him. I stood in the choir feeling as if I were facing the guillotine. I did not sing aloud. The congregation must have been disappointed because the tenor part was too subtle.

Another embarrassment in the choir happened one morning when I was sitting in a choir seat behind the preacher without paying much attention to his sermon. I was told that there was an emergency call from the hospital. I had to walk out in front of the congregation. I asked Margaret if I could resign from singing in the choir. She persuaded me not to quit.

I did not make as many friends in St. Stephen's Church as I did in the Campus Chapel in Ann Arbor, but I had lunch with Margaret and her friends in a restaurant after the Sunday service. It was good for me that in this church life on Sunday I forgot, at least temporarily, about the hard life of my residency. I found in Margaret a good listener to my grumbling and a good consultant for my problems. She not only listened to my complaints but also encouraged me with her good humor and positive advice. Sometimes she took me in her Chevrolet to Washington Park and we walked in the International Rose Garden, Shakespeare Garden and Japanese Garden. Multnomah Falls was another favorite place we visited on Sunday, driving a long way along the Columbia River. It cured my fatigue and depression due to the hard work in the hospital.

The happiest weekend trip was a drive to the Pacific Coast. Marie and Makiso were with us. We left Portland at noon on the last Saturday in April. After driving two hours we saw the water of the Pacific. The Oregon coast is beautiful, with ever-changing views. Some of the shapes of pine trees reminded me of Japan. The view from the top of a cliff was exactly the same as the view of the western coast of Amakusa Island, located southward across the strait from the Nagasaki Peninsula. Giant rocks stood out in the ocean, and big waves steadily approached from the blue water of the Pacific toward the beach below and then crashed onto the sand and rocks. A splendid view. The coast of sand and rocks extended to the south endlessly. Calfornia must be at the southern end of the coast in the mist. The air was neither too cold nor too warm. I saw sea-birds flying up the sky in the fragrant, sweet air of the spring. The Oregon coast is marvelous. Looking at this view, we ate our lunch and fruit, sipped coffee, and then took many pictures with the ocean in the background.

We drove south until we reached Cannon Beach, the most scenic sand beach on the Oregon Coast. A rock in the shape of a big hood stood near the beach. Pieces of driftwood were scattered over the white sand, but there was no litter on this wide beach. I was tempted to run around on the sand barefoot, enjoying the grandeur of nature unchanged for many thousand years. There were no houses here.

There was a house not far away, however. A friend of Margaret's had a house near Cannon Beach. It was a summer cottage style house in which lived three retired sisters. The 73-year-old eldest sister had been the Dean of the Mayo Nursing School. Another sister was the widow of a physician. It looked like a scene in a drama, when I saw the sweet, gray-haired sisters living together in a chic seaside house looking over the Pacific Ocean. It was a heart-warming sight. No shadow of misery or senility. I envied them. Was it possible because they were in the United States? Or was it the result of their long, hard work and efforts? Anyway, the sisters welcomed us and treated us with hospitality.They spoke elegant Minnesotan English. They were shining old ladies without a shadow. They were actually not old. Their hearts were young and vivid. The great nature of this beach must have kept them young. Daily walks on the beach breathing ozone-rich air must have made them healthy and happy.

After leaving this Garden of Eden, we stayed in a rental beach house. Margaret and Marie cooked a meal, using the food they brought from Portland. After the good dinner we sang together many songs and enjoyed the evening. It was a long day in a strange world. I could not sleep in the bed next to Makiso's.

I felt the need of my own car after coming back from our pleasant drive to the Pacific Coast. If I had my own car, I would not have to depend on Margaret's car. I would have more freedom to go wherever I wanted to go. It costs me 50 cents on the bus and three dollars by taxi to go downtown. The purchase of a used car would save some expense. I decided to buy an old car after obtaining my driver's license. When I told Nicolson about my idea, he answered. "I am leaving for the East before long. You can use my old car. You pay me 50 dollars if you want to have the car."

I accepted his kind offer. His car was an old one, but a big car. Fifty dollars meant 18,000 yen at that time. One could not buy a car in Japan for that amount of money, but it was enough to buy a used motorcycle.

I had to practise driving to get a driver's license, but I had no time for a driver education course. I watched and studied Margaret's driving but needed hands-on experience. I must practise driving myself. Margaret arranged personal driving lessons for me. A teacher came from a driving school in a specially built teaching car on Sunday afternoons. One lesson for two hours costs me ten dollars. I took two lessons, and applied to take the State Driver's License test. I thought the driving test was easy in America, but my presumption was wrong. I passed the paper test but not the practical test. I took the test twice but failed both times. The cause of my failure was that I neglected to turn my head enough to look behind before turning my car to the right or left. I learned too late that the State of Oregon was very strict in issuing a driver's license. Margaret encouraged me after each failure, and I tried again. I passed the test after the third trial. Margaret and her friends gave a congratulation party at a restaurant near the Columbia River. Nicolson left for the East as soon as he received the fifty dollars.

He might have paid even less than fifty dollars for this ancient rattletrap, named Henry, when he bought it in the first place.

A new resident of neurosurgery came in July. My new roommate was Jack Sinclair, with dark hair and dark eyes. He had a muscular body and did not speak much but looked reliable. He would not run away like his predecessor, who could not tolerate the life of neurosurgical residency. Now I could enjoy freedom every other night. We were on duty in turn. If necessary, he could request the help of the chief resident. I had to teach him all about the resident's work in neurosurgery at first, but he was quick to learn. By the end of the first month he was able to manage every minor duty of a resident. Dr. Austin took a vacation in July and August. I had to substitute for him. A clinical professor helped me in major surgery, but I had a busy summer with Jack. It was the last week of August when I was allowed a week of vacation.

Margaret recommended that I go to Ashland to see the Shakespeare Festival. A German girl called Christa wanted to go with us. At the last moment, Margaret told me she could not go. I took Christa in my old "Henry" and we started for Ashland.

This travel was a series of troubles. After starting from Portland early in the morning, we had a flat tire before the car reached the Oregon Coast. I had never changed a tire before, but Christa helped me. We started again but I was uneasy. We drove down the Oregon Coast to the south at slow speed. It was the evening of the next day when we arrived at Ashland.

“The Merchant of Venice" was playing that night at the outdoor stage of the Shakespearean-style theater. I had not read the play, but I enjoyed it because the pronunciation of the actors was clear with British accent, and I knew the story. Songs accompanied by the lute were soft and elegant, conjuring up, as if by magic, the Elizabethan Age. I was glad that I came to Ashland, because I had not expected to see a genuine Shakespeare play in the United States.

The second trouble happened on our way home. We intended to go back to Portland after stopping at famous Crater Lake surrounded by the Sierra Nevada mountains. The road became rough and tough as my "Henry" ran from Ashland to the uplands round the Sierra Nevada. The air was dry, and green was rare. "Henry" panted on the winding, uphill road, puffing up boiling steam, like a hot spring fountain, from his nose. He stopped moving at last because there was no more water to cool his overheated engine. What could I do on this high mountain road under the scorching sun? Christa and I looked at each other in dismay.

We sat on the roadside and waited for someone to help us. Half an hour later, a truck approached us. It stopped before we shouted at it. The driver saw that we were in trouble. He came out of the truck and listened to our story.

"Leakage of water from the radiator must be the cause. I have something to fix it." He took out a bottle of fluid from his car and poured it into the radiator. Then he went to find water. After a while he came back with a bucket of water and filled the radiator.

"This will do for a while." he told us, and left with a wave of his hand as we tried to thank him. He looked like "a Buddha met in Hell," as a Japanese idiom says.

Thanks to this truck driver, we finally arrived at Crater Lake and experienced its deep, mystic quietude. Looking down the blue, serene water from the steep edge of the lake I marveled at the grandeur of the American native landscape and the wonder of the kind American spirit alive in the truck driver.

The third trouble with "Henry" occurred after we came back to Portland. I was invited to dinner at the home of a grey-haired lady who worked in the Medical Library. I led her to the back seat of "Henry," and we started from the Medical Library in the evening. On the downhill road, "Henry" rolled too fast, and I tried to control the speed by stepping on the brake pedal. The brake did not work! I tried a few times without success. I clutched the hand brake and pulled it as hard as I could. The car slowed down slightly but kept running down the hill. I saw the red light in the crossing road at the foot of the hill. My "Henry" will crash with another car in a few seconds! I looked at my lady through the back mirror. She sat there peacefully without realizing the peril ahead of us. Gripping the hand brake tightly, I froze in terror. No one saw my pale face, but I saw the glowing red light ahead. "This is the end!" I ran across the intersection under the red light. I thought I was dead, but I was not. No car collided with my "Henry." It was lucky. "Henry" stopped at the roadside after running several meters past the crossing. My desperate grip on the hand brake helped stop the car. Thank God I did not kill this sweet old lady.

# 16

# ELECTRO-ENCEPHALOGRAPHY (EEG)

"Henry" was a cheap 50 dollar car, after all. The owner of a gasoline station advised me, "The cost of repair will be much more than the price of this car. It would be better if you bought another car." He sold me a used car for 100 dollars. It was larger than "Henry," and looked better than "Henry."

But I was too busy to enjoy driving a car. Jack Sinclair was a good resident and helped me, but the final responsibility was on me, the chief resident. Besides, there were operations every day in three hospitals including the Hennepin County Hospital next to the Medical School Hospital. The Veterans Administration Hospital (VAH) was located a few blocks away from the Medical School Hospital. The car saved my traveling time. I drove to the hospital every day since I was assigned as the chief neurosurgeon to the Veterans Administration Hospital. I was glad that I had my driver's license.

The capacity of beds in the neurosurgical wards of the VAH was only twenty, but many more patients were sent from private clinics. The number of inpatients doubled at last. I refused to admit any more patients, because general practitioners continued to send us patients who were unable to pay their bills. Dr. Austin had warned me not to take patients who would not pay the fee for surgery. My decision made the Supervisor of the hospital mad. He suddenly fired me on September 24 on the ground that I drove away the poor war veterans from the Veterans Administration Hospital.

Dr. Austin was embarrassed, but he understood and ordered Jack to work at the VAH. I resumed my work in the Medical School Hospital and the Hennepin County Hospital. I became busier than before. In addition to daily surgery, every intravenous infusion and change of the urethral catheter of male patients were my responsibility along with angiography, schedules for surgery, explanation to patients and their families, consecutive surgery, post-operative observation, prescriptions, orders to nurses, tape recording of surgical notes, changes of dressing, and checking of medical records. Nearly no time for rest. Answers to the daily requests for consultation cases had to be given within 24 hours. It was after midnight when I finished my examination of the referred patients and description of my impressions and recommendations. I took a short sleep until 6:30 in the morning, hoping no emergency would disturb my sleep.

I often wondered whether I should give up my training in neurosurgery. I was not sure if I had enough physical strength to continue this tough daily life of residency. Another anxiety was the uncertain possibility of practising neurosurgery at the University of Nagasaki. The main interest of the Second Department of Surgery had been abdominal surgery. I had succeeded, fortunately, in introducing and teaching pulmonary surgery, but no one in my department had been interested in neurosurgery. Would our Professor and Associate Professor support me if I became isolated from the majority in the department? Neurosurgery cannot be done single-handed, even if it does not need a large team, as heart surgery does. I had no confidence in my ability to practise and develop neurosurgery in my own medical school successfully. It might be wiser to study anesthesia, to start a department of anesthesiology in Nagasaki. I might be wasting my time and energy here in Oregon.

I did not, however, switch to anesthesiology. My classmate, Shigeru Hatano, wrote me of his intention to study anesthesiology at Northwestern University in Chicago. He would become the good anesthetist our medical school needed. I had to keep studying neurosurgery to contribute to our school in Nagasaksi. It was true that I had critical moments when Dr.Austin blamed me for mistakes or when I felt my work was too much. I stayed because I had no money to buy the flight ticket, but another good reason was the presence of Margaret, a kind, helpful friend.

While I was struggling with diarrhea, despair and disappointment, the year 1958 was coming to an end. The total number of surgical cases for this year was nearly 600, a high-ranking figure for one institution in the United States. Now Dr.

Austin trusted me more, scolded me less, and no longer interfered with my work. He even praised me. When I asked him to let me go home at the end of the first year, he insisted that I stay one more year to help him in the laboratory and to study other aspects of medicine related to neurosurgery. I followed his advice because I was anxious to study more, even though Miwa was waiting for my early return to Nagasaki.

There was no Christmas vacation for a resident. I was allowed to attend the midnight service on December 24 and to have Christmas dinner with Margaret and her friends on December 25, because Margaret had negotiated with Dr. Austin. On all other days I kept working until the end of the year. There was no New Year Holiday in America.

New staff members arrived in January. Dr. Ross, who came from the East, was appointed as Assistant Professor. Dr. Jackson came from the University of California in San Francisco, where he had been a resident of neurosurgery during the last three years. He was younger than I but had longer experience in neurosurgery. He was a big, muscular man who behaved as if he were a veteran Army doctor. I worked with him only in the latter half of January. After February I was free from the clinical work.

As I expected, Margaret arranged a sukiyaki party at her apartment and congratulated me on my achievement in clinical neurosurgery. I had not, however, anticipated Dr. Austin's invitation to his home party to thank me for my hard work. He invited not only all the staff and their families but also Professor and Mrs. Roy Swank of Neurology and Professor and Mrs. Weis of Surgery. He presented me with a fine briefcase and a book by Harvey Cushing, *The Pituitary Body and its Disorders*. With this appreciation and recognition he wiped away all my accumulated unhappiness and complaints.

My study in the Department of Neurology started in February. I went to the office of Professor Swank, asking for his guidance. He replied. "You may rest today. We will begin tomorrow morning." What a difference from the Department of Neurosurgery! Besides Professor Swank, there were Dr. John Austin and Dr. Janice Stevens in the Department of Neurology. I did not see Dr. Engel, a German scholar, who worked in the Pediatric Department to study the brain waves of children.

I planned to study electro-encephalography, first. Dr. Stevens was in charge of the EEG laboratory. She was a brilliant neurologist who had recently attended an international EEG meeting in Moscow representing the U.S.A. I felt uneasy when Dr. Stevens looked at me with her big, dark eyes set on mine. She spoke in a brisk, sharp way, and then waited for my answer in silence. It made me nervous, until I realized gradually that it reflected her sincere personality and her eagerness to educate a resident from Japan. I studied hard to respond to her expectations. She did not use any make-up on her face, but she looked attractive when she smiled, with dimples in both cheeks. She knew how to encourage me.

My job was to interpret the daily EEG records. Dr. Stevens checked my reports and corrected my mistakes. In a sense, I was tested by Dr.Stevens every day. It was not hard work but a continuation of mysteries and puzzles. I was affected by Dr. Stevens' enthusiasm, and concentrated on this new study of brain waves. Months passed fast, and Dr. Stevens found fewer mistakes in my reading of EEGs. She was pleased with my progress, and I became confident with my interpretation.

Christa was an EEG technician, as I wrote before. She helped me and encouraged me all the time. She was happy about my improvement in EEG study, too. Dr. Stevens invited us to her home together. But Christa preferred the home of Dr. Engel, because they could talk in German. Also, she often took me to the home of her uncle. These visits with him gave me a good opportunity to learn German conversation. I tried to understand their German and speak German myself as much as possible. Christa was a daughter of a German pastor and after the death of her father she came to Portland, where her uncle and Dr. Engel lived.

Once a week I attended the conference of neurologists. And there was also a joint conference with neurosurgeons and neuropathologists. These conferences kept me busy, but gave me opportunities to absorb new knowledge and learn new approaches to problems. I felt the need of further study every time I listened to discussions in the conference. I visited the Medical Library more often. Margaret helped me whenever I needed a specific book or journal. Books were not enough to learn neuropathology. "Brain cutting" was another duty of mine. I went to the Department of Pathology and dissected many brains. It was very difficult to remember all anatomical terminology of the brain. It was far more difficult to make correct diagnoses of the pathological changes in the brain. This difficult work, however, helped me later, because success with the qualiifying test for a neurosurgeon depends much on the knowledge of neuropathology.

Every Saturday I worked in Dr. George Austin's laboratory assisting him with his experiments. My work was to open the skulls of African monkeys and insert EEG terminals into their brains to record the brain waves. The theory, purpose, and plan of the experiments were all in the mind of Dr.Austin. I operated and maneuvered as he ordered me without knowing why. It was not fun, but I had to do it, because he paid me fifty dollars a month for my work in the laboratory. I pleased him when the result was satisfactory, but I also displeased him with my mistakes and failures. This work had to be done very carefully. If a monkey died during an experiment, it cost Dr. Austin a considerable amount of money to import another monkey from Africa. Unfortunately a few monkeys died after my operations, and I felt miserable each time.

Nevertheless, Dr. Austin appreciated my work, and gave me permission to attend the American Congress of Neurology in Los Angeles. To save money, I traveled on the Greyhound Bus and enjoyed the grand view of the States of Oregon and California on the long bus ride to Los Angeles. I met the Yoshida family again in Los Angeles after a five year interval. They had moved to California from Minnesota while I was in Japan. Mr. Utaro Yoshida was now eighty years old and Mrs. Yoshida was seventy-five years old. They welcomed me with tears in their eyes. Their daughter Kuwa was the widow of a Chinese who died shortly after their marriage; she was now working at a hospital to support her parents and her jobless brother. I appreciated the hospitality of this humble family. Kuwa took me in her car to show me the beautiful streets of Los Angeles and the scenic Santa Monica highway, with impressive, big palm trees on both sides.

The Neurological Congress was instructive for me, with its pre-congressional seminar in addition to many lectures and presentations. A few Japanese scholars reported their studies in English, but they often misunderstood questions and could not follow discussions. It is not easy for a Japanese to join discussions in English.

When I came back to Portland, I was surprised by the news that Dr. Stevens had broken her leg on the previous Sunday when she was skiing. I had to take responsibility for making all EEG diagnoses. Four days later, I saw Dr. Stevens in a wheelchair wearing a plaster cast. It took more than a month before she started her routine again in the EEG office.

Dr. Stevens suggested to me that I should stay another year in her office. Dr. Swank, the head of the Department of Neurology, also promised to pay me 300 dollars a month if I remained in the department. A famous hospital in Portland also proposed to pay me 6,000 dollars a year for research work in neuropathology. I thanked them, but had no choice but to turn down all offers.

It was difficult, however, to refuse the offer from Dr. Austin. He insisted that I should stay to continue my work in the laboratory, because his projected experiments were making good progress. He thought I should stay with him until a university offered me a position of Professorship. It was tempting, because I had no guarantee to be promoted in Nagasaki University, and I knew that neurosurgeons were treated and rewarded well in the United States. Yet I could not accept the offer. Dean Professor Koyano and Professor Tsujimura wrote me letters asking me to come back to Nagasaki without delay. My stay in the United States was too long for Miwa, who had been waiting for my return to Nagasaki for nearly two years. I decided to go back to Nagasaki in September via Vancouver.

Shortly before my departure, Margaret was admitted to Providence Hospital for treatment of her sciatic nerve pain. Surgery on the nerve was performed on August 28 by a neurosurgeon whom I knew. I assisted him in the operation. The surgery ended, but the pain persisted. When I visited Margaret on the day before my departure, she was still on medication to relieve her pain. It was hard for me to leave Portland when she was still in pain. I wonder if I could have stayed as a resident of neurosurgery without her help and encouragement. I owed her so much, yet I did not pay her back anything. I thanked her and apologized, but she told me, "You don't have to pay me anything. Please, help others as I did." I found in her an example of a "good Samaritan."

# 17

# "BEN CASEY OF NAGASAKI"

I started neurosurgery in Nagasaki as a lonely pioneer without the title of professor. In spite of my anxiety, more and more neurosurgical patients were referred to me, and I found opportunities to operate on difficult cases including brain tumors. One reason for the good start was the cooperation of young staff from other departments, but there was another help. It was a television program called "Ben Casey," which started when I came back from the United States. Ben Casey, a young, earnest neurosurgeon, struggled to help and save his patients under many difficult situations in this TV drama. It became a highly popular TV program. Everyone was attracted to the hero. Before long I was nicknamed "Ben Casey of Nagasaki." People learned in this program that a neurosurgeon can save severe cases of head injury. It became a new faith and people no longer hesitated to undergo surgery in the cranium. This new trust in neurosurgeons contributed to the increased flow of neurosurgical patients to my clinic.

1960 was the year when motorization in Japan speeded up further. I bought a second-hand small automobile called "Subaru," a popular product of Fuji Heavy Industry Company, and enjoyed the speed and convenience. It was no wonder that traffic accidents increased everywhere in Japan. The number of victims reached the highest post-war record in 1961. More than 80 percent of deaths caused by traffic accidents were due to head injuries. It was the era when the need for neurosurgeons was realized by the general public.

As a consequence my work became extremely busy. Many young surgeons of the Second Department of Surgery were attracted to neurosurgery and wanted to become neurosurgeons. They were Drs. Jiro Moroki, Shigeyoshi Teramoto, Hirohisa Ono, Mituo

Kaneko, Shobu Shibata, and Haruo Kitajima. All of them have succeeded in their new speciality after many years of hard work. Other young surgeons in the department were also assigned to treat the neurosurgical cases in turn, and they learned gradually how to treat them and how to assist in neurological surgery. My classmate Dr. Shigeru Hatano came back from Northwestern University after mastering anesthesiology. He started in Nagasaki as the head of the Department of Anesthesiology with the help of Dr. Yutaka Goto, who learned general anesthesia with me in earlier days. Their contribution to neurosurgery was remarkable. We can concentrate on our work on the brain and spine.

Head injuries caused by traffic accidents look awful sometimes, but they are not as dangerous as they appear, if the patients are alert. Compound fracture of the skull can be treated surgically without leaving obvious scars. Depressed fracture does not require surgical operation unless it is deep enough to cause neurological deficit. Foreign bodies which stuck into the head must be removed surgically, of course. I remember a high school student who was struck on his head by a sharp wooden bar carried on a passing truck. The piece of wood hit his head and penetrated his skull. No functional disturbance was left after surgical removal of the long piece of wood, because it slipped over the dura, the thick membrane to protect the brain, and did not damage the brain or the brain vessels. Another interesting case was a hunter who shot himself in the head while he was checking his gun. The unexpected blast of the gun drove a bullet into his skull through the forehead. He was carried to a hospital in Shimabara. I drove in a hurry to the hospital from Nagasaki, and successfully removed the bullet from his head without leaving any dysfunction. I knew that he would survive because he did not lose consciousness until I arrived.

The dangerous type is the one in which the consciousness deteriorates without big wounds on the surface. It is a sign of progressive swelling or bleeding in the brain. Correct diagnosis and quick intervention are urgent. Epidural hematoma means bleeding from the arteries on the surface of the dura. If surgery is delayed, the patient cannot be saved. Prompt action is required. I remember a case in the Isahaya Prison. After a fight between two prisoners, one of them became unconscious. I was called in. After seeing the patient I suspected bleeding inside the skull. He was brought to the

University Hospital and operated immediately to stop his bleeding, just in time. He was saved. If one found a linear fracture of the temporal bone, one should suspect bleeding of the underlying artery, but bleeding can start without fracture, making the diagnosis difficult. The change of consciousness is a key to the diagnosis.

Acute subdural hematoma is the bleeding from the veins rather than the arteries under the dura, often at the top of the brain. Therefore, the speed of losing consciousness is slower than in epidural hematoma, but it is often accompanied by edematous swelling of the brain as a result of contusion. The patient may die of severe edema even after removal of the hematoma. The diagnosis of acute subdural hematoma is not difficult, because the patient becomes unconscious shortly after the head injury. Misdiagnosis is, however, frequent in chronic subdural hematoma in which the symptoms appear much later when the memory of the head injury is nearly lost. The complaint of headache might be treated as common chronic headache, and mental confusion would be diagnosed as arteriosclerosis or mental disorder. Not a few of the subdural hematoma patients died in a mental hospital.

Near the end of 1960 a 29-year-old man was referred from the Nagasaki City Hospital for examination of his headache of unkown etiology. He was struck on the head at the annual Nagasaki Festival called "Okunch" in October. His headache started one month later and persisted. He was admitted to the City Hospital for examination, but the doctors could not find the cause of his headache and decided to send the patient to the University Hospital.

An angiographic study of the brain vessels was done on the following day by injecting special dye into the carotid artery at the neck immediately followed by x-ray photographing of the head. The angiograms disclosed compressed arch of the arteries over the brain. It was nothing but a subdural hematoma. It had accumulated slowly after the trauma, but headaches did not occur till one month later, confusing the doctors who did not suspect the one-month-old trauma as the cause. The patient was scheduled to be operated on the next morning.

The patient was still drowsy when he was moved back to his ward after angiography. I thought that anesthesia at the time of examination had been too strong. Nevertheless, I telephoned the nurse at night and asked how this patient was. She answered, "He is sleeping well." A few minutes later, she phoned me, "But he is not breathing."

I jumped up and ran to the ward. It was too late. He was dead. The nurse thought he was asleep, but the pressure of the hematoma mass reached to the medulla oblongata and stopped his breathing.

I realized the seriousness of chronic subdural hematoma for the first time. I regretted that I did not remove the hematoma as soon as I had found it. It was my mistake that I planned to operate on the next day. The textbooks of neurosurgery recommend immediate removal of chronic subdural hematoma.

Since that sad experience, I tried to remove any chronic subdural hematoma as soon as I found it. In the earlier cases I opened the skull by removing a bone flap above the hematoma and took out the hematoma with its membranes. In the later cases, however, I made two burr holes in the skull and washed out the hematoma and its membranes, as described in the textbook written by Dr. G. F. Rowbothum of England. The result was much better than I expected. The time needed for surgery was short. No complication occurred. No recurrence of hematoma symptoms appeared. In those days other neurosurgeons in Japan were practising the standard craniotomy as performed in the Tokyo University Hospital on chronic subdural hematoma, and postoperative infection and convulsion were often reported. In my trephination technique, the time needed for surgery was much shorter, less than half an hour, and no postoperative complications followed. As I reported on my experience of 35 cases of chronic subdural hematoma at a neurosurgical meeting, neither death nor complication followed the 27 cases of trephination surgery, while one of the earlier cases of craniotomy died.

Another unfortunate case was a one-and-a-half-year-old boy. He was wrestling with his brother at home and hit his head when he fell on a tatami mat. He was not wounded, but a few days later he vomited and became semicomatose. Angiographic examination revealed subdural hematoma. Craniotomy was performed immediately to remove the entire hematoma mass from his brain. The surgery was successful but his temperature went up and he died at midnight. The cause of death was lack of fluid, a basic mistake in fluid-intake control. Chagrined by this experience I learned the importance of fluid administration in children too late to save this poor child.

One half of the causes of chronic subdural hematoma was traffic accidents. The rest were caused by other types of head trauma. There were some cases of unknown etiology. Epileptic seizure was suspected as a cause in some. Repeated hitting of the head at a low ceiling was suspected in another. A friend of mine, a family physician, complained of chronic headache. I discovered that he had chronic subdural hematoma and removed it, but he had had no experience of earlier accident except a fall from a horse more than twenty years ago during the war. He is still alive and practising in Nagasaki, almost twenty years since his hematoma was removed.

The former Mayor of Isahaya City was another case of unknown etiology. This fine gentleman developed unusual behaviour and was diagnosed as senile dementia due to arteriosclerosis. After admittance to a local hospital he became drowsy, and I was consulted. I suspected chronic subdural hematoma and confirmed the diagnosis by angiographic study. He was brought to the surgical theater of the hospital immediately and the hematoma mass was removed. After regaining full consciousness, he confessed that he threw his head against a wooden pole in his house several times in despair after he lost his beloved wife. He survived and at the age of 92 he is still living in Tokyo with his daughter.

Chronic subdural hematoma can be treated without difficulty by simple drilling of burr holes in the skull, a happy procedure for a neurosurgeon. I also remember a case in Omura. The patient was an old physician. He was diagnosed as having a stroke, and his consciousness went down constantly. I was consulted by a surgeon in the Omura City Hospital. By questioning his family I found out that he had recently fallen from his bicycle on the way to visit a patient. I suspected subdural hematoma, and confirmed my diagnosis by cerebral angiography. The hospital did not have neurosurgical equipment but I dug out surgical instruments applicable to neurosurgery and conducted surgery on hematoma under local anesthesia. In the course of the operation the patient regained consciousness as the hematoma mass was removed from the brain surface, and started talking and moving. We had a hard time to keep the patient quiet until the surgery was finished. When he came out of the surgery room, he surprised his family and relatives, who thought he was a ghost, because they were ready for the funeral and were discussing how to divide his properties among them. He resumed his practice soon and has been well ever since.

I must confess that I was once helped by a patient with chronic subdural hematoma. One day in Nagasaki I was caught by a policeman for violating the speed limit. When I was walking down the stairs of the Urakami Police Station after submitting my driver's license, a policeman with a white helmet stopped me. "Hello, Dr. Kawano. What happened? Why are you here?"

I wondered who he was, looking at him on the dark stairs. Then I remembered that he was a policeman who had developed chronic subdural hematoma after hitting his head at a *kendo* (Japanese fencing) match, and was operated at the University Hospital. I explained why I was there. Before the end of my story he told me, "Wait here for a moment, please." When he came back he had my driver's license with him. He laughed, "If a neurosurgeon does not have a driver's license, it will be a disadvantage for us patrol policemen who must handle traffic accidents."

Unfortunately this was the only time he helped me in my frequent violations of the speed limit, which was too slow for a neurosurgeon.

By 1969 I had experienced 60 cases of chronic subdural hematoma in ten years. The result was far better than in other institutions, as I reported at a Japan Neurosurgical Society Meeting and published in a medical journal.

# 18

# *ABC* SYNDROME

Chronic subdural hematoma is not a common after-effect of mild head injury. Neither palsy nor convulsion will follow mild head injury. The most frequent complaint of many victims of simple head injury is the so-called post-traumatic headache with additional complaints of pain in the shoulder, arm and hip, dizziness and sleep disturbances.

These patients request x-ray study and EEG examination, which usually fail to disclose any abnormality. Neurological examination will confirm normal functioning of the central nervous system. Yet the patients insist that something must be wrong after head injury, and ask for hospital care. If they are refused admission to a hospital or further examination, they go to another clinic or hospital requesting examination and treatment. The symptoms are the typical syndrome of "indefinite complaints." They will be satisfied if a doctor gives a diagnosis of "dysfunction of the autonomous nervous system," believing it to be certification of post-traumatic damage to be financialy compensated. Doctors prefer this vague term to post-traumatic neurosis or hysteria, although the definition and pathology of this dysfunction are not clear.

However, it was no longer a joke as the so-called "whip-lash injury" following a smash of a car from behind became a big topic in the mass media. It was argued that headache and neck and shoulder pain in these cases persist because of the pathological changes of the neck caused by the striking force of a car colliding from behind. Some orthopedic surgeons reported abnormal EEG in these whip-lash injury patients. Others theorized that damage to the parasympathetic nervous system in the neck is the cause of all the ambiguous symptoms of the head, neck and shoulder. As a neurosurgeon I could not be silent, because no EEG abnormality was proved in the so-called "whip-lash injury" cases as well as in the "post-traumatic syndrome" patients. Orthopedists in Keio University Hospital also reported that the EEG of whip-lash injury patients was normal in nearly all cases. Interpretation of EEG is not easy, as I found at the University of Oregon. Even if one discovers an abnormal EEG in those post-traumatic patients, it is too soon to judge it to be the result of injury, because more than five percent of healthy medical students revealed abnormal EEG in the tests at our medical school. How can one conclude that the abnormal finding in an EEG is the result of an automobile accident without comparing it with an EEG recorded before the injury? Such a conclusion would be misleading and unscientific.

In response to mass media reports of whip-lash and other traumatic injuries, I started a study of post-traumatic headache. Among 428 post-traumatic patients of mine there were 290 patients (63 percent) who complained of headache longer than two weeks after head injury. More than 80 percent of those chronic headache patients had cooled their head with ice bags or cold towels after head injury. It is possible that cooling of the head could reduce blood circulation in the cooled scalp and the involved nerves such as the great occipital nerve and trigeminal nerve, reducing their tolerance to pain sensation. I asked Dr. Shobu Shibata and Dr. Goichi Matsumura of our department to check the electron-microscopic change of the nerves of rabbits after cooling with ice. As a result of the cooling, the degeneration of mitochondria was demonstrated in the nerve cells, suggesting a lowered pain threshold. However, the chronic post-traumatic headache could not be explained by cooling of the head alone. There must be other factors.

I next reviewed the duration of bed-rest after injury. The average bed-rest of 215 head injury cases was 23 days, more than three weeks. It was too long for simple head injury, even though 111 cases lost consciousness temporarily after injury. The longest bed-rest without any wound or surgery was 220 days. The average of 24 so-called whip-lash injury cases was 68.8 days, and the longest was 522 days, without any fracture of the skull or neck.

Another surprise was the difference in the length of bed-rest between the "self-injury" and "non-self-injury" patients. The average of the former was 15.7 days, but of the latter was 28.3 days. The longest record belonged to the "non-self-injury," of course.

What is indicated by these figures? The physicians would not order such a long bed-rest. It must be by the request of patients who regarded the bed-rest as "necessity" or "advantage." If the head injury is caused by another's fault, then the victim of the accident has the right to get compensation. The amount of compensation is usually calculated by the degree of incapacity resulted and the length of hospital care. If no abnormality is found on physical and radiological examination, the length of hospitalization is the only measure to decide the grade of compensation. The amount of compensation will increase as the patient complains of various symptoms and stays longer in hospital or continues to visit a neurosurgical or orthopedic clinic. This type of patient refuses to leave hospital, insisting on the need for further treatment, even if the doctors recommend discharge. Some doctors would not insist upon discharge, because the longer stay of the patients is profitable for the hospital. They yield to the plea of the patients to stay.

On the other hand, those "self-injury" patients who can blame no one but themselves for their injury, do not have the privilege of getting compensation. They want to go home and work again as soon as the doctors permit them to leave the hospital. No wonder the "self-injury" group's bed stay is shorter.

For many years in Japan the major cause of death had been tuberculosis of the lung, which needed a long bed-rest for treatment. Therefore bed-rest became a golden rule for any illness. A common expression of visitors at leaving the bed of a patient, "Please, take good care," meant good and long bed-rest. The patient hesitates to leave the hospital bed.This hesitance will be increased when visitors tell him about the cases of later development of post-traumatic disorder as the result of neglected treatment and bed-rest. The attitude of the patient's family is much kinder after head injury than before, particularly when the patient is in a hospital bed. It is convenient and comfortable for the patient, if not necessary, to stay in bed longer.

In general, Japanese people believe that one must stay in bed after hitting one's head. Everyone regards bed-rest as necessary to avoid the after-effects of head injury. The patient himself becomes nervous and anxious if he is not staying in bed. Therefore he continues to stay in bed.

There is a simple method to test the grade of anxiety. It is called MAS(Manifestation of Anxiety Scale). As soon as I learned that this test was used in the Clinic of Psychosomatic Medicine, Kyushu University, I ordered many MAS testing sheets, then compared my patients with normal subjects, randomly selected. The result was interesting.

Only one of 12 normal controls revealed anxiety (8.3%), whereas 23 of 26 post-traumatic chronic headache patients (88.4%) exhibited unusually high anxiety. Another contrast was between the "self-injury" and "non- self-injury" patients, 27.8 : 85.0%. What does this mean?

The "self-injury" patients have no reason to worry about compensation. On the other hand, the "non-self-injury" patients think about compensation and are often not satisfied with the proposed amount of compensation. Consciously or unconsciously they prolong their stay in bed to increase compensation. The longer they stay in the hospital, the more they worry about home and work. Anxiety increases, and sleep at night becomes shallow or disturbed. Lack of sleep and lack of exercise weaken the muscular strength of patients, and they gradually develop lumbago or shoulder and arm pain. After lying for a long time in a horizontal position, the neck muscles to support the head become weaker and easily get tired and painful in a sitting or standing position. The patients believe that these muscular pains must be the after-effect of head trauma and jump into bed again. The vicious circle continues and the patients lose their chance to get up and work. To end this vicious circle, they must use their muscles and train them for daily activity and work in spite of the pain. The patients neglect this effort because of anxiety and greed for compensation. Doctors must help the patients to remove their anxiety, but many do not understand or accept this responsibility, or are reluctant to persuade the patients to leave, so they let them stay in the hospital. This delays rehabilitation of the patients. The word "rehabilitation" means "going home" in Latin. No wonder that the patients with "post-traumatic syndrome" increase endlessly. I coined a new name, "ABC syndrome," for this vicious circle: "A" for anxiety, "B" for bed-rest, and "C" for compensation. I explained the mechanism of this vicious circle to the patients, removing their anxiety and encouraging them to overcome it and to go back to their home and their work.

# 19

# LOMA LINDA, CALIFORNIA

Professor George Austin left the University of Oregon and became a professor at Loma Linda University. He asked me in a letter to work with him as a Research Fellow. I agreed and I arrived at Loma Linda on June 2, 1968, after visiting Professor G. R. Nunn of the University of Hawaii and his family in Honolulu and revisiting Portland, Oregon, and then staying three days in Sausalito, California.

Loma Linda means "Lovely Hill" in Spanish. This small university town in the San Bernardino Valley is surrounded by desert. The only small hill I found was the one near the Loma Linda University Medical Center. It did not look "lovely" to my eyes, which are used to seeing Japanese hills and mountains, although the green color of the few trees contrasted with the white, dry sand. The town of Loma Linda, however, was clean and sanitary. Not a single piece of trash was to be found on the wide street. I saw people walking only occasionally. Traffic was sparse. The only big building was the ten-story building of the University Medical Center. Flat one-story houses without fences stood on both sides of the streets. Sprinklers were shooting water onto the green lawns. The only store I found was a supermarket selling general goods, but no tobacco or coffee was sold, because the town belonged to the Seventh Day Adventists. There was only one shop where one could drink coffee and eat meat. It was a small restaurant in front of the motel where I stayed on my first night in Loma Linda. "Heathens" use the restaurant, but no Adventist will go there. After experiencing the strange taste of soybean hamburger in the Medical Center, I decided to eat once a day in this small restaurant, disregarding the disapproval of the townspeople.

The Medical Center was a beautiful, new building. The spacious, elegant lobby surprised me as soon as I entered. I found the office of Professor Austin as refined as the lobby. The clover-shaped four wings of the hospital were designed beautifully and efficiently. The ICU (Intensive Care Unit) had a nurse station in the center surrounded by see-through single rooms, a clever design enabling the staff to watch patients all the time. Smoking is prohibited in the whole building, and smokers must smoke somewhere outside the hospital, although I seldom saw smokers. More than 90 percent of the employees and patients of the Loma Linda University Medical Center were Seventh Day Adventists, nonsmokers.

Fortunately I found a room for rent in a newly-built house on the day after my arrival. When I visited an office near the hotel in order to look for a room, I happened to meet Mrs. Brooks, who was looking for a tenant. She kindly suggested that I live in her house. I followed her advice without hesitation. It was a new house without much furniture. The room for me was a handsome sleeping room. A large new bed had been brought in before I came. One of the walls was a large mirror, and the floor was covered with a thick, green carpet. The bathrooms had no bathtub but a shower system. The room was worth the rental price of 65 dollars a month. Mrs. Grace Brooks had been in England for six months with her eleven-year-old daughter. I did not ask her about her husband, but later I learned that he had died of a brain tumor six years earlier. Mrs. Brooks looked stern, but she spoke British English, which was easier for me to understand than American English.

Robert Kennedy was assassinated on the day after my arrival at Loma Linda. People were upset and daily activities were slowed down even in Loma Linda for a few days. It was one week after the event that the subject of my research was given and I started experiments. Professor Austin seemed excited about his model of cerebral circulation, but the work he assigned to me was not so dramatic. My assistant was Bill Hayword, a Catholic and a smoker, a non-conformist in Loma Linda, but we worked together all right. He was a nice fellow and a good partner. After eating breakfast at the infamous coffee shop near the Health Center, I worked in the laboratory until noon. I found a nice place to spend the whole noon hour. It was a swimming pool on the medical school campus. The daytime air of Loma Linda was hot even in June, often over 100°F. I enjoyed the pleasure of diving into the cool water after running over the hot, burning earth. The pool was free of charge. No one else was around at lunch hour. Swimming was an enjoyable exercise during my monotonous research life in Loma Linda where I had no acquaintance except Dr. Austin, a critical teacher. People in Loma Linda stop working on Friday afternoon. Even if one wants to work, it is impossible because everybody else goes home. I gave up and went home to take a nap in my room, which had no table or chair.

There was no place of entertainment in this community. A supermarket and a drugstore were doing business, but the only coffee shop-restaurant closes its door at three o'clock in the afternoon. I had no place to eat supper. At five o'clock, however, Mrs. Brooks told me that I had an invitation for dinner from her neighbor, Jean Neufeld. Jean, a Britisher born in London, welcomed us at the door. Her husband, Roland, was a Canadian architect. His brother John, a dentist, was also invited. I was introduced to their daughter and two sons. The girl paid no attention to me, but her younger brother was curious about this Asian stranger. Their grandmother arrived at last. She was a tall, graceful lady. At the dinner no meat was served in this vegetarian home, but the atmosphere was nice. The brown buns baked by Jean in the morning were delicious. Following the dinner there was merry, pleasant conversation. Jean's father is a pastor who moved from London after the family settled in California. All the family started hymn singing accompanied by Jean's piano. I enjoyed singing with them. At the end of singing Jean stared at me with her shining, blue eyes and told me, "You sing beautifully. Please, join in our choir and sing with us." I accepted her kind offer with pleasure, although I had no confidence in my singing in a choir.

The next day was Saturday, the Seventh Day. The Adventists do not regard Sunday as a holy day. Saturday is the Sabbath Day for them, as it has been for Jewish people since the day of Moses. The Adventists do not work during the holy Sabbath from the evening of Friday to the evening of Saturday. Not only are they different from other Christians in this practice, but also they observe vegetarian rule and refuse to eat meat. Neither do they drink coffee, tea or alcoholic beverages. No smoking at all. Absolutely no work on the Sabbath. The post office is closed on Saturday and opened on Sunday. Mail is delivered on Sunday instead of Saturday. Nearly all the people in town move towards the church just before morning service begins. Jean's car came on time and we went to church with Mrs. Brooks and her daughter.

The church stood next to the University Health Center. Its name was the "University Church." It looked like a big city hall, quite different from the small, humble churches in Japan. Jean took me to the back door of the church and led me to a room behind the altar, exchanging words with every friend she met on the way. She introduced me to the choir conductor. The young conductor welcomed this non-Adventist, non-American new member with a friendly smile.

After a short rehearsal of the hymns for the morning service, we went to the last row of the choir box. I was tense and nervous, because this was my first experience singing unfamiliar hymns in this unfamiliar church. In fact, it was easy. No one noticed my singing in this big choir with a good number of other tenors. Jean sang in her seat for altos, and occasionally looked at me to send me a reassuring smile that said "Don't worry." The songs were new to me, but they were sung beautifully under the good conductor. I was surprised that I became a member of a church choir in Loma Linda the week of my arrival.

The life at Loma Linda University was monotonous, but gradually I became acquainted with the staff and other townspeople and began to enjoy the life in this dry and simple town. Bill was a good assistant, although he was a Catholic and lived in another town called Redlands.

A medical student named Arden visited our department of neurosurgery frequently, with hope of becoming a neurosurgeon. Once he invited me to his house. There was a pool inside his house. All his friends, boys as well as girls, enjoyed swimming in the pool under colorful illumination. I felt uncomfortable in this luxurious house, but I appreciated his attempt to cure my loneliness. Much more enjoyable was a trip he took me on to Sea World in San Diego. I saw the grand ocean of the Pacific and watched the skilled, acrobatic jumps of seals, forgetting the passing time.

I was not the only Japanese in Loma Linda, but the other Japanese were Niseis, second generation Japanese Americans. I was once invited to the home of a Japanese-American professor of psychology. His children looked like Japanese, but they could not understand Japanese. It was a strange experience talking with

Japanese children in English. Nevertheless, I enjoyed the Japanese dishes prepared by the Japanese wife of the professor. It was a happy evening.

More often I visited Jean, nearly every Friday when Jean baked buns and announced on the telephone: "Buns are ready. Come soon, while they are still warm." These visits, besides being pleasurable, gave me a good opportunity to listen to Jean's good British English while we ate the hot buns and sipped the black tea prepared in the British style. As a daughter of a pastor, Jean sang songs well and played piano beautifully. She also was a good reader and a poet. She showed me her poems, and I tried to make poems to show her. I was lucky to find a good English teacher in her, but I felt guilty because I was entertained by her with delicacies instead of paying tuition.

One evening we were both in Redlands to attend an outdoor concert. Jean's parents were with us, for they were also music lovers. The daytime in July was warm with the summer heat, but it became cooler in the evening at the park. We sat on a bench behind the semicircular lines of wooden benches surrounding the stage. A conductor appeared on the stage and urged the audience to practise singing. After the practice, the visitors from other towns were asked to introduce themselves. I told them that I came from Nagasaki, Japan. The audience clapped hands as a sign of welcome.

Finally, young ladies in colorful evening dresses came on stage, followed by young men with bow ties. They joined in singing beautiful songs. I was surprised by the high quality of the chorus and solos. It was much more than small town music. No wonder—there was a school of music at the University of California in Redlands!

More surprising was the performance of Beethoven's “Kreutzer Sonata" which followed. The violin solo of the girl in a scarlet evening dress overwhelmed me; it was much more moving than the music I used to hear on the record player. Everyone stood up to give endless applause. It was amazing to find such a talent among unknown, young musicians. Jean and her parents were as happy as I was that we had come to this concert.

Seeing that I enjoyed music so much, Jean took me to another concert in August. It was in the Hollywood Bowl in Los

Angeles. A Japanese violinist, Miss Masuko Ushioda, played Tchaikovsky's violin concerto with the Los Angeles Symphony Orchestra conducted by Hiroyuki Iwaki. It was exciting for me to listen to the music played by Japanese musicians in the famous and enormous Hollywood Bowl. It was an excellent performance, as we expected. The audience's standing ovation lasted long in the sunset glow of the sky. I gave thanks from my heart to Jean and her twin sister, Doreen Buckwater, for taking me to the concert.

Professor Austin suggested that I stay longer than three months in Loma Linda, but he finally agreed to let me leave Loma Linda for Nagasaki at the end of August. He also wrote for me a letter of recommendation to Professor McNaughton of McGill University, Montreal, Canada.

When the day of my departure approached, I felt sad to leave Loma Linda, which I did not much care for at the beginning, when it seemed a tasteless desert town. By this time, however, I had found another Research Fellow from Japan, Dr. Eiichi Hirai of Nagoya University. He and his wife welcomed me at their home every time I visited them. They were sorry that I was going to leave Loma Linda. Jean did not tell me how much she would miss me after my deparature, but I could see how sad she was. After singing and chatting with me, suddenly she became silent, to my embarrassment. I knew that she wanted to keep me near her longer as a friend and confidant. Therefore, I went with her on my last Sunday in Loma Linda when she invited me to a day tour to Laguna Beach. I thought she would ask Mrs. Brooks to join us, but she did not.

Laguna Beach is on a beautiful stretch of coast south of Los Angeles. Even in summer, not many people were bathing on this beach, as it was too far from Los Angeles. The beach was quiet and peaceful. Jean's main purpose was to show me a small museum, but it was closed on this Sunday. Then, Jean headed her car to a small restaurant near the beach. It looked like an arbor in a flower garden, surrounded by various flowers of many colors. The restaurant was crowded with customers on this last Sunday of August. We had to stand for a while waiting for an empty table. It was amusing to watch lightly dressed, chatting couples in the waiting line and to look around the flower gardens and the blue ocean in the distance.

Our turn came at last, and we were led to a table near the window. The view of the blue Pacific Ocean from this table was marvelous, reflecting the deep blue, cloudless sky of California. We sat there in silence and kept looking at the beauty of nature. We looked at each other occasionally and nodded to each other, saying silently, "Isn't it wonderful? Aren't we happy that we came?"

The lunch was delicious. Jean knew well what was good on the menu, because she had been here many times. When we finished, only a few customers were still there. Soon we were the last customers. The room became quiet. We hesitated to talk loudly. No word was necessary. We avoided mentioning the subject that was most on our minds, knowing that this would be our last time to be together. We were grateful to each other, but we did not need to express gratitude to each other. We knew too well how we felt deep in our souls.

When we realized that there was no one else in the restaurant, we left this unforgettable place and walked to the seaside. There was a long sandy beach between the flower garden and the ocean. We walked and walked until we sat down on the sand exhausted. We watched the sun sinking down into the big Pacific Ocean. The setting was one of unforgettable beauty and serenity.

It was already dark at night when we returned to Loma Linda.

# 20

# MARIA VON TRAPP IN STOWE,VERMONT

A few years before my stay in Loma Linda, there had been an international conference on hematology in Japan. After the conference, Professor Yoshito Takaoka invited Professor Wilhelm Raab to Nagasaki with other scholars as guests to his department of internal medicine. Professor Raab was famous for his works on hormones and many other fields of medicine. He was the co-author of *The Hypokinetic Disease* (1961), which was translated into Japanese. A dinner party to welcome him was held in the Yataro Hotel on a hill overlooking Nagasaki Harbor. I was invited to the party and allowed to sit close to him. When Professor Raab was fascinated by the dreamy evening view of the harbor, Professor Takaoka asked me, "Dr. Kawano, would you sing a German song for Professor Raab?"

After a moment of hesitation I sang "Heiden Roeslein," composed by Werner. Professor Raab listened to the song with his head down. When I finished singing, his eyes were wet. With deep emotion he said, "How could I expect to hear this song, which my mother used to sing for me in my childhood, in this Far East city after so many years!"

He told me how he escaped from Salzburg and immigrated to the United States with the Trapp family just before Hitler marched into Vienna. He also told me that he was teaching at the University of Vermont, that Maria von Trapp, the author and heroine of the "Sound of Music," lived in Stowe, Vermont, and that they visited each other very often. At the end, he insisted that I should come to Vermont to meet Maria. In the next month came a letter from Maria telling me how she was impressed by my article "How I Survived the Atomic Bomb," which I had given to Professor Raab. She was eager to meet me at Stowe, but I was not able to visit her until the fall of 1968, after my stay in Loma Linda,

I left Loma Linda early in September. I arrived at Burlington Airport on September 16, after visiting Chicago, Washington, New York and Boston on the way. Professor and Mrs. Raab welcomed me at the airport. They took me in their car and Mrs. Raab drove the car to Stowe.

It was still summer in Loma Linda and trees should still be green in Japan in this season, but here in the State of Vermont, the leaves of the trees were already changing their colors. As the car drove up the hill, the color of the leaves became rich and the red tone increased. It was a perfect autumn view when we reached Stowe. Suddenly there appeared a Swiss-style hotel with a steep roof and big, dark, wooden walls. Every window was decorated with flower boxes. One felt as if one was transported to Switzerland from America.

Maria was standing on the lawn with her guests. As soon as she saw us, she hurried to us with a happy smile. She was quite different from the image of Maria played by slim Julie Andrews in the "Sound of Music." The real, stout Maria grasped my hand firmly with her big, warm hand.

The name "Trapp Family Lodge" does not fit this big building with a capacity for 200 guests. Stowe is a famous ski resort. In winter the Lodge must be full. Even in this early autumn, nearly every room was occupied. I was allowed to use a room which had been the Trapp family's room for their daughter before her marriage. Maria treated me as a family member instead of a guest. Baron von Trapp had passed away already, and the children were married and had left Stowe. There was left only the youngest son, who was taking care of the Lodge. He looked handsome. His gentlemanly attitude reminded me of his father in the movie.

Maria was quite different. At age 63, she preserved the merry, innocent unpredictability of a girl. Yet she never missed greeting every guest with her cheerful smile. She introduced me to a group of guests who surrounded a table in the lobby. I saw how much she was loved by them all. Her closest friends, however, were the Raabs. They spoke to each other in German with a Viennese accent. I remembered what Mrs. Raab had mentioned quite casually in the car, "I have lung cancer. I don't think I can live any longer than one year."

When she was chatting with Maria, she looked so happy that she did not look like a patient who expected death in the near future. Was she enjoying the last autumn of her life with her dearest friend? Before the sun set, the Raabs said goodbye to us and left for Burlington.

The next day, Professor and Mrs. Raab came again to Stowe. They kindly drove me to Montreal to visit the Desroches, whom I had met earlier in Nagasaki. I was surprised when the car entered Montreal in two hours from Stowe, crossing the border between the United States and Canada so easily. Professor Raab knew the city of Montreal well. The car stopped at the Children's Hospital where Dr. Jean-Marie Desroches worked. Dr. Desroches was waiting for us in front of the hospital. This gray-haired professor welcomed us. It was four or five years since Dr. and Mrs. Desroches had visited the Redemptoristine Convent in Nagasaki. Mrs. Desroches is a younger sister of Mother Marie-Ange, Mother Superior of the convent.

After saying good-bye to Professor and Mrs. Raab, Dr. Desroches took me around the Children's Hospital before going home. At the Desroches home, Mrs. Desroches gave me a warm welcome. While we were talking about Nagasaki, her children came back from school. The eldest daughter was a medical student. The second daughter was studying in a nursing school, and the youngest girl was a junior high school student. All of them gathered in the living room before dinner. It was their custom to sit together in the living room and spend time in pleasant conversation about what happened during the day, before moving to the dining room. Dr. Desroches and I were the only males surrounded by four fair ladies who served us drinks. I did not know what kind of drink I should ask for. One of the girls presented me a glass, saying, "Why don't you try rum and Coke?" I tried it, and it tasted good. Since then, rum and Coke has become my favorite cocktail in Canada. On the third day I met the son of Dr. Desroches. He had graduated from a medical school and was busy at the moment as an intern in a hospital. He brought his fiancee with him. The Desroches family spoke French with each other, but in my presence they spoke English. I missed the opportunity to learn French.

On the next day Dr. Desroches took me to the Medical School of Montreal University, where he taught psychiatry, and then we went to the Montreal Neurological Institute of McGill University. I met Professor McNaughton, a gray-haired gentleman. He introduced me to Professor Rasmussen, the Director of the Institute, and Professor Lukas Yamamoto, a neuroradiologist, and at last to Professor Hanna Maria Pappius, who was famous for her study on brain edema. I was hoping for a position as a Research Fellow at MNI, but the possibility was dim.

After three days in Montreal, I returned to Stowe to spend the week-end with Maria. Professor and Mrs. Raab came from Burlington, too. It was a good weekend. Maria wanted to keep me close to her. On Saturday afternoon we went horseback riding together around the beautiful hills of Vermont. After leaving the horses in the stable, we took a walk to Mansfield Lake. The lake was surrounded by trees with colorful leaves. We walked along a lane by the lake looking at the birch and maple trees. Maria kept talking about her life in America and her concern for Austria and Japan. We had so many things in common: experience of defeat in the War, life in a different culture, love of music, and independent Christian faith of our own. We understood each other as if we had been friends for many years. Maria regretted that she had missed an opportunity to visit Japan in the past. I encouraged her to look for another chance.

After the dinner, Maria again took me outside, and we watched in silence the beautiful sun setting behind the mountain. At the end she held my hands and confided that this day was the anniversary of her marriage to the late Baron Georg von Trapp. I knew how much she missed her husband, who did not live long enough to celebrate their Golden Wedding Anniversary together.

Saturday night is the time for a dance party at the Trapp Family Lodge. As soon as the waltz melody of Strauss started, Maria asked me to dance with her. I hesitated because I could not dance well. Maria gave up and danced and bounced like a young lady with another man. I regretted that I had not learned dancing in my young days. Nevertheless, I was envied by other guests because Maria did not leave me all evening.

Maria's dream to see Japan became a reality within ten years. At the age of 72, Maria came to Japan at the invitation of a

TV station. After appearing on TV in the program called "Tetsuko's Saloon," she took a long trip to Kyushu with her interpreter-friend Ruth Hetcamp. When she landed at Nobeoka, Miyazaki Prefecture, from a ferry boat, she was the same Maria, looking just as she had looked in Stowe. We drove across Kyushu Island in Ruth's car through the Takachiho Gorge, Mt. Aso, and Omura Bay until we arrived at Nagasaki at last. Maria and Ruth kept singing their familiar songs in German all the way in the car, and I joined them whenever I found any familiar melody. I should have recorded them on tape, for they sang so well, and so happily.

Maria went back to Stowe and lived there until she died at the age of 82, on March 28, 1987, ten years after her visit to Japan. A few years before her death, the Trapp Family Lodge caught fire and was burnt down on Christmas Eve. It must have been a heavy blow to Maria. How sad she would have been after losing all her dear possessions, and the documents which connected her to her husband and family! Yet alive forever in my mind is the memory of the days I spent with Maria in the beautiful hills of Vermont.

# 21

# CEREBRAL ANEURYSM

After the weekend, I went back to Montreal again and stayed in the home of Dr. Desroches. No paid fellowship was available at the Montreal Neurological Institute, but even so, I wanted to study at the institute every day. The Desroches family were generous. They not only allowed me to stay at their house but also treated me as a long-staying guest. It was the beginning of autumn in Canada, where the air was nice and clean and the maple leaves were at their best color. If you stand on the hill of Montreal, which means Royal Mountain in French, you would see a dome of McGill University through the maple trees. I did not realize that the laboratory of Professor Pappius was under this dome until I went up to the top floor of the building to help her experiment on animals.

Professor Hanna Maria Pappius is a world-famous biochemist who was born in Poland as a daughter of a diplomat. She laughed when I told her that her first name sounded like "Hana," a popular Japanese name for a woman meaning "flower" in Japanese. She welcomed my offer to assist her in her laboratory, and guided me to the top floor of the modern, hotel-style building which I saw from the hill. My assigned work was to give injections to the experimental rabbits and anesthetize them.

Professor Lukas Yamamoto welcomed me, and wanted to show me his exquisite color photographs of blood circulation in the brain. I imagined his long, hard work and endless study of radiology since he had come to Montreal shortly after graduation from a medical school in Hokkaido. He kindly explained to me the interesting pictures of the brain to demonstrate cerebral circulation under many different conditions.

Since the retirement of Professor Penfield, the founder of MNI, in 1950, Professor Rasmussen succeeded to the position of chief of the Institute. Yet I saw Professor Penfield occasionally when the visiting professors or scholars gave us lectures or participated in staff meetings. These meetings and speeches were valuable opportunities to improve my knowledge and thinking on neurology and neurosurgery. I understood why this institute has been regarded as a "Mecca" of neurosurgery and neuropathology in the world.

More than eighty percent of the residents in Montreal are descendants of French ancestors. They speak French. The language used in the University of Montreal was French, and Dr. Desroches taught there in French and talked with his family in French, but he and his family spoke to me in English. Therefore, the life in the Desroches home did not improve my French at all, but gave me good opportunities for horse-riding. The Desroches owned a large piece of land in the suburbs. To their country house on the bank of the St. Lawrence River belonged a large stable where horses were kept for every member of the family. On Friday evenings, the whole family moved to the country house by car, one hour from Montreal. They took me along as a guest. From the dining room of this big country house I enjoyed the view of the St. Lawrence river with its endless flow of cargo ships.

On Saturday and Sunday we all went out riding. The youngest daughter rode on her pony with amazing skill. I followed her on another horse toward the forest of colorful autumn trees as beautiful as the trees in Vermont. The brightest among the trees was the red Canadian Maple. The shape of the leaf is different from our Japanese maple, but the beauty of the color is the same. Riding through the branches of maple trees I was amazed at the big size of the forest. It took nearly one hour to go through the forest, and I was amazed again when I was told that we were still on land owned by Dr. Desroches. It is an unbelievable luxury in Japan to ride around a large forest of one's own every weekend with the whole family. Even in Canada, where the price of land is much cheaper than Japan, it must be a special privilege allowed only to those who inherited a vast land from their ancestors, and Dr. Desroches must be one of them. Anyway, I was glad that I had such a rare opportunity of riding with them over their land at the height of the Canadian autumn.

The reason why the Desroches welcomed me and treated me so kindly was that I was the medical consultant of the Redemptoristine Convent in Nagasaki. Mrs. Desroches is a younger sister of Mother Marie-Ange, who came to Japan from Canada to open the Redemptoristine convents, first in Kamakura and then in Nagasaki. My relationship with the convent in Nagasaki began when a Japanese Sister became ill.

Several years ago, the young Sister complained of headache soon after her new assigment to an unpleasant job at a regular change of roles in the Convent. A physician of a Catholic hospital was called in. After finding no physical abnormality, this doctor diagnosed her condition as a symptom of hysteria. Mother Superior could not believe the diagnosis and consulted with a neurologist of the University Hospital. Dr. Masaharu Takamori of the First Department of Medicine, one of our neurological conference members, went to the convent and examined the Sister. He suspected subarachnoid hemorrhage due to ruptured cerebral aneurysm, and referred her to me.

His diagnosis was correct. As I injected a radio-opaque solution into her common carotid artery, the series of x-ray shots demonstrated a red-bean size aneurysm at the junction of the internal carotid artery and posterior cerebral artery at the base of the brain. This inborn aneurysm must have ruptured at last after slow enlargement over many years. She survived the rupture because the bleeding was not much, but the problem was how to prevent the second rupture.

At the University of Oregon, I assisted Dr. Austin when he operated on ruptured aneurysm. He ordered me to find out the common carotid arteries and vertebral arteries on both sides and to pass tourniquets around the arteries to get ready to compress the vessels at any critical moment in order to control accidental bleeding from the aneurysm. It was not easy to expose the main arteries which provide blood to the brain arteries, but this precaution could prevent disastrous mass bleeding during aneurysm surgery. After this precautionary maneuver, Dr. Austin opened the frontal portion of the skull and slowly approached the aneurysm in the base, gently compressing the anterior surface of the brain. As an assistant I was nervous, anticipating a sudden bleeding, the worst thing that could happen. Dr. Austin shouted "Damn!" and fought in the depth of the skull to stop the bleeding from the ruptured aneurysm. I was upset but waited patiently for his order to bind the supplying arteries temporarily. Fortunately the bleeding was controlled and the neck of the aneurysm was closed with a metal clip. The long battle was over. Dr. Austin and I were exhausted.

The number of aneurysm procedures in which I assisted Dr. Austin was not many, and none of the patients died after surgery, but I was shocked when I found a report by McKintosh, a British neurosurgeon, on his experience with 772 cases of cerebral aneurysms. Of 385 cases he operated on, 109 cases, or 28.4 percent, died. This mortality was no better than the percentage of death in the non-surgical group, 27.8 percent. I was scared by the risk of surgical treatment of aneurysm. And it was why I hesitated to operate on cerebral aneurysm when Dr. Masaharu Takamori referred to me my first case of cerebral aneurysm in the spring of 1961. The patient was a 56-year-old woman who had suddenly complained of headache and then lost consciousness. Three days later her consciousness came back, but her right eyelid remained closed. When examined, her right eye did not move from its lateral position and her pupil was wide open. The ruptured aneurysm must have compressed the oculomotor nerve. The clever Dr. Takamori had made the correct diagnosis of ruptured cerebral aneurysm and had consulted me.

I decided to occlude the common carotid artery, a much safer procedure than the direct attack on the aneurysm under craniotomy. The purpose of the surgery is to reduce the risk of rerupture by closing the common carotid artery of the affected side, because the closure would lower the blood flow and blood pressure to the aneurysm. I heard once from a professor of otorhinolaryngology that he had often ligated one of the two common carotid arteries at operations on cancer, and no serious effect on the brain had resulted.

I exposed the right common carotid artery of this woman and tightened the ligature gradually, checking on the condition of the patient. The artery was closed completely at last, but nothing happened. Neither physical nor mental change resulted from this surgery. Instead, the oculomotor palsy improved slightly. Her eyelid opened before long, although she could not move her right eyeball. No second rupture occurred since then. The patient was still alive and well at more than eighty years of age. The same surgery was applied to other aneurysm cases one after another. The 31-year-old Redemptoristine Sister was the seventh aneurysm patient for me.

After undergoing the revised operation of common carotid occlusion, this young Sister returned to the convent in good healthy status. Since then Mother Marie-Ange of the convent asked me to come to the convent and see the patient whenever any sister became sick. I became the consultant physician at this Catholic convent of strict order, and freely examined sisters in their rooms. Mother Marie-Ange trusted me completely, and introduced me to Dr. and Mrs. Desroches with complimentary words when they visited the convent in Nagasaki. This was the background of their warm hospitality in Montreal.

According to the Cooperative Study reported by Dr. Sahs' group in 1966, one half of unoperated cases of ruptured aneurysm died within six months and 32 percent of operated cases failed to survive the direct surgical attack on the aneurysm. What interested me most in this report was the result of carotid artery occlusion. Only 21 percent of the cases died of rerupture after this simple technique of common carotid occlusion. It was a wise decision that I, as an unskilled neurosurgeon, performed this simple, safe surgery for my aneurysm patients. My early experience of 25 cases of common carotid occlusion was reported under the title of "Subtotal Common Carotid Occlusion as a Treatment of Ruptured Aneurysm" in a Japanese Journal, *Brain and Nerve,* in January, 1968, before my departure for Loma Linda. After my follow-up of 50 cases of subtotal common carotid occlusion, only two patients, or 4 percent, died within six months after surgery, and 40 patients, or 80 percent, were alive after six years. At that time I was not aware that a new technique to prevent rupture of cerebral aneurysm was in progress in Switzerland.

On October 19, I flew from Montreal to Europe. I stopped in Paris, London, Stockholm, and Stuttgart to visit hospitals and universities. My final stop in late October was Zurich. There was working at the Kantonspital a young Japanese neurosurgeon from Kyoto. He introduced himself as Dr. Haruhiko Kikuchi and kindly guided me around this teaching hospital of Zurich University, but I knew nothing about the skill of his teacher, Professor M. G.

Yasargil, who was operating on the arteries of the brain under the surgical microscope.

Two years later, this Professor Yasargil was invited to Japan for a teaching course in microsurgery. Dr. Kikuchi accompanied him as his favorite assistant and interpreter. I applied for this course and was impressed by the new technique to anastomose, or connect, fine arteries under the microscope. Dr. Kikuchi later came back to Japan, although Professor Yasargil tried hard to keep him in Zurich. He became a pioneer of microsurgery in Japan, and had worked as the chief neurosurgeon at the National Center for Circulatory Diseases until he was appointed as Professor of Neurosurgery at Kyoto University. As soon as he came back to Japan I asked him to operate on a case in Nagasaki. He demonstrated his skill under the surgical microscope which I borrowed from the Department of Ophthalmology. It was the first case of microscopic neurosurgery in Kyushu Island.

The Nagasaki University Hospital bought for me a Japanese surgical microscope and I started to use it for delicate surgical maneuvers. The more I used it, the more I became eager to master the technique under Professor Yasargil in Zurich.

# 22

# THE GUESTS OF *EXPO '70*

The social climate in Japan had been unstable since June 15, 1968 when radical students from Tokyo University occupied Yasuda Auditorium on the University Campus, protesting against the approaching renewal of the Security Pact between the United States of America and Japan. In the end, it required 8,500 armed policemen to drive out the students from this famous University Hall in January, 1969. The Socialist Party and student groups continued their fight against the Pact, causing friction at every level of Japanese society. They also requested that U.S. occupation of Okinawa be ended. It was the World Exposition '70 started in May, 1970 at Osaka which brightened the atmosphere of Japanese society.

Sixty-four million people including many foreigners visited this big-scale exposition by the time the exposition closed on September 13. One of them was Lore Walb from the Bavarian Broadcasting Company, Munich. When she came to Nagasaki to meet German Sisters in the Franciscan Convent, Dr. Akizuki of St. Francisco Hospital asked me to help her as an interpreter. I took her around Nagasaki, showing her the Atomic Bomb Memorial Museum and other famous sightseeing spots in the city. She was thrilled when Miwa and I took her to Unzen National Park and stayed overnight in a Japanese inn with a big hot spring bath. She enjoyed everything so much that she revisited us before leaving for Germany. We drove to Amakusa Island in my small car, enjoying the breathtaking view of the coast and the sight of potatoes growing in roadside potato fields. At the time of farewell, she insisted that I should come to Munich and visit her in her apartment house.

Another unexpected guest of Expo '70 was Christiane Eckert, a granddaughter of Dr. Albert Schweitzer. Her mother, Rhena Eckert, was the only daughter of Dr. Schweitzer. Rhena came to Nagasaki in April, 1963 on a speech tour arranged by Asahi Press, and I happened to be her interpreter on the stage of Nagasaki City Auditorium. My interpretation of her speech was appreciated by the audience, including Dr. Nomura, who worked with Dr. Schweitzer in Lambarene, and by Dr. Koyano, President of the Nagasaki Schweitzer's Friends Society, because of my correct translation of medical terms. Together with Rhena we went to Unzen for an overnight stay. Rhena was given a suite in the Miyazaki Inn and Dr. Nomura and I stayed in the Unzen International Hotel.

The next morning, when I visited Rhena at the Miyazaki Inn, she welcomed me to her suite and we enjoyed talking with one another. She treated me as if I were her old friend, and I did not feel that it was my first meeting with her. After all, she was the daughter of my spiritual teacher, who changed my course of life. We found that we had so many things in common, our way of life, our thinking and philosophy. We were also close in age, only one year difference, and were born in January, as Dr. Schweitzer was. We understood each other, and felt the happiness of free, warm communication. We knew she had to leave in a few hours and we would miss each other thereafter.

Hurried up by Mr. Tokutaro Kitamura, a member of the National Assembly, Rhena came out of her room and stood at the entrance of the hotel. To my surprise, she refused to ride with Mr. Kitamura in the waiting American car. Instead, she got into my small Subaru. Mr. Kitamura disclosed his irritation, but Rhena ignored him and sat next to my driver's seat. Mr. Kitamura gave up and rode in the big car with Dr. Nomura. "I wanted to talk with you a little longer," explained Rhena as soon as our car started and added, "I also wanted to try this tiny car."

If the president of Fuji Heavy Industry Co., who produced this beetle-style car smaller than the Volkswagen, heard her remark, he would have felt honored.

The drive from Unzen to Tahira Port was not long enough for us, as we had so many topics to talk about. The green golf course on the slope of Mt. Unzen and the winding roads overlooking the blue Ariake Bay did not interest Rhena, who kept asking about me and about my experience of the atomic bomb in Nagasaki. We arrived at the port of Tahira too soon. Rhena had to step up to the ferry. On the deck she waved her hand for a long time after the ferry left the shore

Seven years after our meeting, her second daughter Christiane came to Nagasaki to see me. She was one of four grandchildren of Dr. Albert Schweitzer, and she loved music. Her father, Mr. Eckert, was a pipe organ builder born in France. She started her piano lessons at the age of four, and went to the Zurich Conservatory at age sixteen to study piano and pipe organ for four years. However, she became interested in medicine after staying in Lambarene every summer and helping her grandfather's work with her mother, a medical technician. She was twenty-two years old when she entered the Medical School of Lausanne University. The next September, her grandfather, a theologian, an organist, a saint of Lambarene, the philosopher of "Reverence for Life,"closed his 90 years of life. Then Christiane moved from Lausanne University to Zurich University. She not only studied medicine but also took piano lessons from Madame Irma Schaichet, a good friend of Rubinstein as well as Dr. Schweitzer. She used every spare minute for medical and piano study.

In her last year of medical school she planned to get more clinical experience at St. Luke International Hospital in Tokyo before taking the final examination of her medical course. Shortly after she arrived in Japan she came to Nagasaki to see me at her mother's suggestion.

When I met Christiane for the first time, she was a tall woman, 28 years of age. The color of her hair was light brown, and her big shining eyes were almond. Her innocent smile was charming. Her English had a French accent but was good and fluent. Her manners were gentle and polite. She cared for Miwa, who welcomed and loved her as I did.

She stood for a few minutes in awe when I took her to the tree her mother had planted seven years earlier in front of the monument near the hypocenter of the atomic bomb. She visited the Atomic Bomb Memorial Museum in Urakami and the Glovers' house in Oura with keen interest, but what appealed to her most was the view of Omura Bay from a beach north of Nagasaki. In the afternoon of late August, "Pearl Bay" was quiet and peaceful without any other bathers. The only visible building was a hotel on a cliff. Wearing nothing but a bathing suit Christiane and I walked on the sand into the sea. We started to swim slowly toward the center of the bay. When we felt tired, we returned to the beach to lie down on a flat rock under the sun

Christiane enjoyed the peaceful view of the sea and the quietude of this seaside much more than I did. She felt all the dust and fatigue of her long trip from Zurich to Tokyo disappear completely. She lay there for a long time with a happy smile on her face, looking into the distance filled with serene blue color.

After staying five days in our house, she went back to Tokyo for her clinical training. She wrote to me from Tokyo that she wanted to spend a month in Nagasaki at the University Hospital. I asked Professor Takaokato to give her an opportunity to study in his department of medicine. He agreed, and I wrote to tell her the good news. At the end of September she moved from St. Luke International Hospital to our house in Nagasaki. For four weeks she went to the University Hospital and shared the ward round and clinical discussion with other staff and students in the First Department of Internal Medicine until October 25. I introduced her as my friend, not as granddaughter of Dr. Schweitzer, to protect her privacy. She enjoyed her daily experience in the University Hospital, and she also enjoyed the life in our home. She was always willing to help Miwa in the kitchen. She liked to cook and proved her skill in cooking. We enjoyed the delicious taste of her cooking. She taught Miwa how to cook special curry rice flavored with pineapple and paprika. It became my favorite menu in our home. The two women in the house communicated with each other using Japanese and gesture language, because Miwa could not speak English. This turned out well for Christiane, because she learned good Japanese through Miwa quite naturally. She made good progress in Japanese by the time she left Nagasaki at the end of October.

Christiane missed Japan after her return to Zurich. She asked me often in her letter to give her an opportunity to have a piano recital in Nagasaki. As a member of a volunteer group called "*Usagi-kai*" (Rabbits Club) I was active in helping four orphanages in Nagasaki. After consultation within this group, we finally decided to have a charity concert. The Nagasaki Symphony Orchestra was more than happy to play with Christiane, the granddaughter of Dr. Albert Schweitzer. They needed the support of members of the Kyushu Symphony Orchestra and recommended Mr. Takeichiro Yasunaga as the conductor of the concert. After being introduced to Mr. Yasunaga I asked for his help. He agreed to conduct the orchestra for Christiane. The concert was scheduled for the spring of 1972, six months after Christiane's graduation from medical school, to allow her enough time to practise for the concert.

It was my first experience in organizing a concert. Gradually I realized how difficult it was to prepare for one. I had to beg for support from various people and groups. I designed and edited the concert program. I had to work hard to sell as many concert tickets as possible through many friends and volunteers. The members of Nagasaki Symphony Orchestra and the members of "*Usagi-kai*" kindly cooperated with me. When I saw the finished print of the concert program with a large photograph of Christiane playing the piano on the front page, my heart was filled with emotion. The order of the music was arranged by Christiane:

Schumann: Thirteen Children's Scenes
Mozart: Piano Sonata, C-Major, KV330
J.S.Bach: Partita, No. 1, B-Major
Beethoven: Piano Sonata, No. 14, C-Minor
op. 27-2 "Moonlight"
Mozart: Piano Concerto, No. 12, A-Major, KV414

Comments on each piece by Dr. Nakamura of Yamaguchi Prefectural Hospital were added on the following pages.

After passing the national examination of the medical board and after practising each piece long enough, Christiane came to Japan on April 5, two years after her last visit. On the next day she was already in Nagasaki, and we met again in excitement and happiness. Soon she started her practice on our piano. She played with the Symphony Orchestra four times before the final rehearsal under the baton of Mr. Yasunaga. She became tense and nervous as the evening of the concert approached.

On the evening of April 14, the concert was held at the Nagasaki City Auditorium. Christiane appeared on the stage with a smile. Her figure was elegant but her piano performance was much more elegant and refined. The audience was fascinated by her music as soon as Schumann's "Children's Scenes" started. Loud applause burst forth after the last tone of Beethoven's “Moonlight” sonata. After the intermission, orchestra members came onto the stage and Conductor Yasunaga stood in front of them. Christiane sat before the piano. Then quietly she started her favorite piano concerto by Mozart. The music had the delicate brilliance of stars in the midnight sky and then sprang to a storm of sounds of harmony.

Listening to the changing modes of this exquisite music, I thought of the late Dr. Albert Schweitzer, who would be thrilled to listen to this music by his granddaughter if he were here. By this evening I returned something to him as a token of my gratitude to him, to whom I owe so much of my career and philosophy. I watched the audience around me with satisfaction. Everyone was spellbound by the marvelous performance of Dr. Schweitzer's granddaughter.

# 23

# MUNICH

For more than ten years I had worked as a neurosurgeon in the University Hospital, but my position still belonged to the Second Department of Surgery, for there was no independent department of neurosurgery at Nagasaki University. It was a handicap. I stayed as an associate professor of surgery, while the chief of the Department changed from Professor Tsujimura to Professor Hirai, and then to Professor Tsuchiya. Tokyo University and Kyoto University had their own departments of neurosurgery already in prewar days. An independent department started in Kyushu University after the war, and yet there was no department of neurosurgery in Nagasaki University until 1972.

Shortly after Christiane left Nagasaki in 1972, the Ministry of Education approved the opening of a new department of neurosurgery in Nagasaki University. It was too late for me. I was already 54 years old when the new professorship of neurosurgery became available. Many candidates were recommended from many universities. I was one of them, but the probability of my appointment was low. I began my career of neurosurgery on my own decision, and studied in the United States without any recommendation by our medical school. In the past ten years I worked as the only neurosurgeon in Nagasaki, without much help from other members of the department. It was an extremely busy life, too busy to indulge in research or laboratory work. My medical publications were not many, except a number of clinical studies and case reports, insufficient for a candidate seeking a professorship. The bigger problem was my age. Only eleven years were left before my retirement age of 65. Some insisted that I should be elected as the first professor of neurosurgery because I was a pioneer of neurosurgery in Nagasaki University, but I anticipated the appointment of someone from Tokyo University or Kyoto University, which had established departments of neurosurgery a long time ago.

As I predicted, Dr. Kazuo Mori, Associate Professor of Neurosurgery at Kyoto University, was elected as the new Professor of Neurosurgery of Nagasaki University. He was a young neurosurgeon around forty years of age. He had graduated from Kyoto University, alma mater of Professor Tsuchiya, the head of the Second Department of Surgery. I knew that Professor Takaoka, a graduate of Tokyo University, helped Professor Tsuchiya in the selection of the new professor. I was offered sympathy, but I accepted Dr. Mori's appointment as a natural consequence. It gave me a good chance to study in Europe, as I had wanted to do for years.

My main purpose was to study microsurgery under Professor Yasargil at Zurich, but I needed to improve my German before going there. I remembered the encouragement of Lore Walb to come to Munich. There was Professor Kurt Decker teaching neuroradiology at the University of Munich. I planned to study neuroradiology in Munich before moving to Zurich. This would be a good opportunity to become fluent in the German language and to make my study of microsurgery easier. Professor Decker approved my application to study neuroradiology in his department. I had to pay all expenses, but I would be able to manage for a short period of three months in Munich. I delayed my departure until the end of October, because it was the year of the Olympic Games in Munich and I had no intention of watching the Olympic Games.

Lore Walb was waiting at the Munich Airport for me and took me immediately on a tour of the Tyrol. Fortunately there had not yet been any snow that year in the Tyrol. The red Volkswagen ran under the clear November sky from Munich towards the North Tyrol city of Innsbruck, the center of North Tyrol, the second oldest city in Austria. It was not big but it was beautiful. I understood why Maria Theresa loved this small city. We took a ride on a trolley car climbing up Mt. Fungenberg, and enjoyed the grand vista of Alpine mountains from a snow-covered peak.

Lore was a wise traveler. She selected a small inn in a suburban village. After dinner we walked to the graveyard behind the village church. Every tomb was decorated with fresh flowers and candles.

Stone angels and Mary the Holy Mother stood smiling among the tombs. Each tomb had the name and the picture of the buried person. I stood in silence and awe in this impressive graveyard in the cold evening of Tyrol. Lore told me that this was All Saints' Day when people visit the graves of their beloved ones.

The following day was another sunny day. It was a continuation of the thrill and excitement to drive on the long, snow-covered mountain road, crossing the Alpine passes one after another, until we finally reached Bolzano, a center of South Tyrol.

The next morning we walked around this medieval town with its old Bishop's palace and cloister. It was a quiet, lovely town. I wanted to stay longer, but we left for Breno, another Tyrol town, where we had the last night of our unforgettable Tyrol tour.

The Neuroradiology Department of Munich University was in a building on Beethoven Street. It was the headquarters of Professor Kurt Decker. Indoors, the old building was poorly illuminated. It looked gloomy, but had the familiar atmosphere of an old university with statues of famous professors from the past. Professor Decker welcomed me with a big gesture and a smile. He suggested that I eat breakfast with him. Ignoring my hesitation, he walked out to a small restaurant where he often ate. I was surprised when he toasted me with beer at this early hour of the day. Was it a custom in Munich to have beer for breakfast? Anyway, he seemed to enjoy his Munich breakfast. As soon as we returned to the Neuroradiology Department, he showed me the latest model of the tomographic x-ray machine which he had designed for pneumo-ventriculography and Philips Company had constructed. I was then introduced to his Associate Professor, who was a stern-looking man, quite a contrast to Professor Decker. Other members of the staff were more friendly and polite.

At five o'clock in the afternoon, Professor Decker called all the staff to a room where wines and food were set on a table. It was a small welcome party for me. Professor Decker was joyous. Everyone ate cheese with wine. I was not used to cheese. Besides, some of it smelt awful. After one touch of it, I could not remove the strong odour from my finger. I confess, however, that the wine was delicious, as it should be in Germany.

The sun rose late in the November morning and sank early in the afternoon in Munich. Every morning I walked on the dark street to a street car station from Lore Walb's apartment, which was located near Nymphenburg, an old summer residence of the Bavarian King at the western end of Munich. It took twenty minutes by street car to reach Beethoven Street. The darkness had disappeared by the time I arrived at the University, but it came back already at four o'clock in the afternoon. I had to walk back to Lore's apartment house again in darkness. The length of daytime became shorter and shorter every day. I felt depressed in the gloomy interior of the Neuroradiology Department during the day. Snow did not fall often, but having snowed, it stayed long on the streets. Dirty snow on the pavement became frozen and I slipped often even with a new pair of snow boots. The coldest time was when I waited for a streetcar at the square in the morning. My fingers ached even in the thick gloves. I stumbled on the frozen pavement. I regretted that I had come to Munich in winter.

There was, however, compensation in the Munich winter. It was the season for opera and concerts. There were concerts nearly every evening. Opera was performed every evening in three opera houses. The biggest was the National Bayern Opera House in the center of the city. It was ruined by an air raid during the war, but was reconstructed in its old prewar style. Even in this opera house where Bavarian King Ludwig II used to come, a ticket for a seat on the seventh floor under the ceiling was surprisingly cheap, although one had to wait in a long line to buy this cheap ticket. Several times I waited there patiently and found friends among the regular fans. Once I found a music-loving Japanese in this line. I cannot forget the satisfaction I felt when I grasped my ticket after a long wait.

I went to the National Opera House and other concert halls often, taking full advantage of the cheap tickets available to students. I was grateful for the opportunity of listening to the performances of famous singers, musicians and orchestras, in spite of certain obstacles I faced. One hardship was the walk to the theater in snow, when others were arriving in their cars. Another problem was the time of the performance, starting at eight in the evening. I am an early riser and become sleepy in the evening. Once I fell asleep in the middle of a long aria from "Tristan and Isolde." Probably I was the only one in the audience who slept during this loud opera by Richard Wagner.

In the front seat of the "Ceiling Box" on the seventh floor one can see only half the stage. Nevertheless, I enjoyed "Aida" and "Tosca" from this "Ceiling Box." This experience in Munich made me hesitant to buy the expensive opera and concert tickets in Japan.

A music loving student informed me of a free concert. It was in a big church near Lore's apartment house. On one cold evening in December I had the privilege of listening to Karl Richter playing Bach's organ music in the church at no charge.

The subject of my research assigned by Professor Decker was the change of the size of the cerebral ventricles by aging. Atrophy of the brain advances as one gets older. And the ventricles enlarge as the brain substances become smaller. If the average size of the ventricles at each age could be found, the abnormal size of a ventricle or the grade of brain atrophy could be easily expressed in figures. My work started with the measurement of all ventriculograms in the department. The main target was the size of the anterior horn of the lateral ventricle. The size of the widest part of the anterior horn was measured on each film and the figures were sorted according to age. Abnormal, pathological brains had to be excluded on the basis of individual case histories studied. Reading the German medical record was not easy, even though my only aim was to find out whether the cases in question suffered from any abnormalities or disease.

From early morning till late in the evening, I kept reading patients' medical records and measured their lateral ventricles. This daily work improved my speed in reading German and increased my knowledge of many diseases. I was afraid that three months was not long enough for this meticulous study, but I finished all my work by the end of the third month. I wrote an article on my study in English and presented it to Professor Decker just before I left Munich. He was satisfied with my work and introduced the article to a publisher. It was printed later in a journal of neuroradiology.

Lore had a senior position with the Bavarian Broadcasting Company, and was already approaching retirement. Her friends were mostly elderly people. Whenever she was invited to a dinner, she took me with her and introduced me to her friends, old ladies living alone in apartment houses. We seldom visited a home with a married couple or children. The reason was that Lore herself was not married. Like many others in her unhappy generation, she lost most of her male classmates in the war, including the boy friend she had wanted to marry.

I did not intend to stay long in her apartment house. I accepted the offer of one of her rooms as a temporary lodging until I found a place to live in Munich. Nor did Lore intend to keep me long; she did not ask me to leave, however, because I was no nuisance to her. Against my intention I stayed for three months in a small room of her big apartment house. She sometimes kindly cooked meals for me. One evening looking at cheese on the dining table, I murmured, "I dislike cheese. It smells awful."

Since then Lore never ate cheese while I was in Munich. I felt sorry for her. On the other hand, I cooked Japanese meals nearly every evening for her, since she appreciated the good taste of the rice I cooked. That was why I never went to a Japanese restaurant in Munich. I did not waste money on eating in restaurants, because lunch was served free at the University. Lore refused to accept any payment for the room and food. Obviously she wanted to repay me for my hospitality in Nagasaki. I thanked her for her kindness.

Near the end of the year, Lore caught cold and could not leave her bed. Her close friend came every day to take care of her. I tried to help her as much as I could, and she appreciated my being in the same building. After New Year's Day she recovered gradually. Near the end of January she invited me to the "Swan Lake" ballet at the Opera House. Our seats were in the balcony, a good place in the center of the lower floor, on which I used to look down with envy from the "Ceiling Box" on the seventh floor. It was close to the special guest box, in which I saw the Japanese Ambassador and his wife. They noticed us and saluted us. Probably they thought I was a rich Japanese who invited an upper-class lady from Munich. I enjoyed the music and dancing of "Swan Lake" that evening much more than I had in the past.

# 24

# ZURICH

It takes only four hours to go to Zurich from Munich, less than the time needed to go to Tokyo from Osaka. I did not realize the existence of the international border until I was asked to show my passport on the train. The officer looked at the passport and me. Without a word he went to the next passenger. My eyes went back to the view from the window again. The evening view of Lake Constance was magnificent. I could not keep my eyes off it until the sun sank completely.

Christiane was not at Zurich Station when the train arrived. After I had waited for some time, she appeared in a hurry. "I am sorry, I had a difficult time to find a place to park my car," she apologized. She had driven from a hospital in Aarau where she was working as a doctor. On our way to a boarding house she explained to me how busy she was in the hospital. She also told me that all expenses in the boarding house were to be paid by her mother, who was divorced from Mr. Eckert after the death of Dr. Albert Schweitzer and now was living in the United States with her new husband, a doctor.

The house we arrived at was the home of Mr. and Mrs. Maurer. Their two daughters had left home after marrying, and one of their rooms was provided for me. It was not a boarding house but the residence of a lawyer. They allowed me to use a cozy room at the request of Madame Irma Schaichet, their neighbor and piano teacher to their daughters and Christiane. Mrs. Maurer was born in Italy. She welcomed me and treated me kindly as if I were a member of her family. She was a typical Italian lady with a warm, happy personality. We had no problem in communication, because she spoke English well.

Christiane introduced me to Madame Schaichet next door. She was a Hungarian and a close friend of Rubinstein. I expected a stern, gray-haired piano teacher, but she was a gentle old lady. She welcomed me as a friend of her beloved pupil. She could not speak English well, and I had to depend on Christiane as interpreter. Madame Schaichet knew that I loved music, and that I had arranged a concert for Christiane in Nagasaki. She suggested that Christiane play a piano piece for me. They sat together in front of a piano, nodded to each other, and then started a duet composed by Bach. Suddenly the gentle, bent figure of an old lady disappeared. In her place was a professional pianist, Irma Schaichet, with a straight backbone and vivid spirit, swaying her whole body in accord with the melody of the music, as if she were in a dream. I remembered the story which Christiane had told me before. Irma Schaichet often complained that people embarrassed her by treating her like an old woman, while she herself always felt young. The beautiful piano music came to an end. Madame Schaichet returned to her old lady role. She served us tea and cakes, saying, "How nice to play with you again like this! You should come to me more often, even though you are very busy." She was in her late seventies, and yet she kept giving piano lessons to young people nearly every day. One of her pupils was a daughter of Professor H. A. Krayenbuhl, a world-famous neurosurgeon.

On the next day I visited Professor Krayenbuhl in the Kantonspital, the teaching hospital of Zurich University. Professor Krayenbuhl stood up in his room to welcome me. He was a gray-haired, tall gentleman with erect posture. He looked much younger than his retiring age of seventy. I presented him the recommendation letter from Professor Decker. When I told him that I had met Madame Schaichet on the previous day, he said laughingly, "My daughter must be a burden to Madame, because she is slow in her progress with the piano." Then he added, "I am going to operate on a brain tumor. Why don't you come over with me to the operating room?"

Professor Krayenbuhl solemnly changed his dress to a surgical gown and approached the surgical table. Without a word he picked up a surgical knife and incised the scalp, which was shaved, disinfected, and covered with clean linen. His assistants clamped the cut ends of the scalp with clamps to stop bleeding from the wound. The exposed skull was drilled with a hand drill to make four holes. A wire saw was passed between two holes and the bone was divided, and then a bone flap was raised. The tumor under the dura was exposed. Without a word Professor Krayenbuhl worked on the tumor, detaching the mass from the brain tissues, clipping and cutting the fine blood vessels which connected the tumor with the brain. The whole procedure reminded me of the methodical tea ceremony. The room was very quiet. Everyone was silent. The professor moved his hands skillfully to follow the set procedure he had practised hundred of times on brain tumors. No hesitation. No confusion. Confidence and fine technical art filled this surgical theater. Bleeding from the vascular meningioma was miraculously controlled under his command. All blood vessels surrounding the tumor were coagulated and divided before taking out the total tumor mass with minimum blood loss. I was overwhelmed by his skilled performance, and admired this veteran neurosurgeon who had worked at his speciality for nearly fifty years, developing new techniques and writing many books on neurosurgery. It was true that he was a great authority in Europe on this field of medicine. When the procedure ended, he turned to me and smiled as if he were asking me "Wasn't it a good operation?" Then he left the table, leaving the rest of the work to his assistants. He walked out of the room as quietly and solemnly as he had entered before the surgery.

In this Kantonspital there were three neurosurgeons from Kyoto University studying neurosurgery. The successor to Dr. Kikuchi was Dr. Yasuhiro Yonekawa, who later became a professor of neurosurgery in this Kantonspital, a new favorite disciple of Professor Yasargil. Dr. Yonekawa was busy taking care of visiting neurosurgeons from many countries. I was one of them and he took special care of me. He knew that I had been the only neurosurgeon in Nagasaki University until Dr. Mori, a graduate of Kyoto University, came as the chief of the new department. Dr. Yonekawa was a nice gentleman. I understood why Professor Yasargil was fond of him and trusted him. Every morning I watched the microsurgery of Professor Yasargil on human brain arteries. In the afternoon I practised microsurgery in a large laboratory where I worked on a carotid artery of a small animal under the surgical microscope.

A large surgical microscope was hung from the ceiling of the surgical theater. It had two scopes for the assistants beside the main scope for the chief operator, to let the assistants see what was going on in the deep field of surgery at the bottom of a brain. There were special stools on which surgeons can operate in a sitting position to reduce the tremor of manipulating fingers. Otherwise, the room was not different from any other surgical theater. An anesthetist put the patients to sleep, one after the other, in two surgical theaters. The anesthesia was maintained by anesthetic nurses in each room. The observation gallery, separated from the surgical theater by a large glass window, was filled with visiting surgeons and medical students by the time the surgery started.

Suddenly silence held the gallery. Professor Yasargil entered the surgical theater. After saying a few words to the assistants, he began the surgery. It was not easy to watch the operation over the shoulders of the audience in the gallery, but I saw how quickly Professor Yasargil cut the scalp, removed a small bone flap and opened the dura to disclose the brain. At this point Professor Yasargil stopped his maneuver and looked up at us and pointed at a brain artery and a meningeal artery to be anastomosed with the brain artery. Then he pulled down the hanging surgical microscope. The audience shifted their eyes towards the big white screen. An enlarged image of the vessels and the tips of a pair of forceps appeared on the screen. As we watched, the blood flow of the two arteries was blocked temporarily by fine clips, and the two cut ends were sewed up with microfine sutures to form a new anastomotic route. It was an extremely difficult maneuver to connect the two arteries of only one millimeter in diameter. The fine suture was thinner than one tenth of a millimeter. When the suturing work was completed in a breathtaking few minutes, the blocking clips were removed slowly to confirm the free flow of the blood through the anastomosed vessel. At the site of anastomosis, minor leakage of blood was found, and softly compressed by a cotton pad. After a while the leakage stopped, The bloody surface of the brain was washed with warm saline solution many times, and then the closure of the wound began. The dura and the scalp were closed in less than twenty minutes. It was a swift, clean and skilled procedure, all done by Professor Yasargil himself. I sympathized with Dr. Furuse who stood there holding the spatula throughout the surgery performed by the professor. Fortunately the length of all operations was far shorter than I expected, only one hour, instead of several hours needed for other neurosurgeons. Professor Yasargil explained to us the details of the surgery while he was waiting for the next patient to be prepared for operation. All explanation was in English, because the visitors were from many parts of the world and were not used to the German language.

The microsurgery of two patients finished by noon. Admiring the perfect skill of Professor Yasargil, I went to the dressing room to change my clothes. When I walked out of the room I was stopped by a woman who had been watching the surgery a few minutes ago in the gallery with us. She asked me in German, "Would you tell me what the Professor told us?" "Where do you come from?" I asked her, because I thought she was a woman doctor. "I am a medical student at this university, but I could not understand him, because he explained everything in English." I was surprised, but interpreted for her in German as much as I could. You could see how international was the fame of Professor Yasargil and how well he treated his visitors in his surgical theater. A big privilege of a Fellow was the lunch at the hospital. A full course dinner was served by waiters in a dining room for doctors at a price much cheaper than in other restaurants. There was a free service of wine in a carafe. I enjoyed eating in this dining room with other Japanese doctors. The lunch hour was long in Europe, and all we had to do in the afternoon was to practise microsurgery in the laboratory under the supervision of Dr. Yonekawa. We used the lunch hour in full and relaxed in this dining room before going to the laboratory. In the laboratory there was no language barrier because we all spoke Japanese. We took coffee breaks often as soon as our eyes got tired of looking at the enlarged figures of small arteries through the lenses of the microscope.

The winter in Switzerland was as cold as I had expected. The downhill slope from the Maurers' house to the street where I caught a streetcar was frozen and slippery in the morning. On sunny days I walked to the hospital all the way. Stores were already open in the early morning and many pedestrians shopped on the way to their offices. I found a bookstore on the street and bought the German texts of *Fuer schlaflose Naechte* (For Sleepless Nights) and *Glueck* (Happiness) by Karl Hilty, the famous Swiss scholar and saint, whose books influenced me since I found Japanese editions of them in my young days. Gradually I was accustomed to the daily life in Kantonspital. I responded to the Zurich morning salute "Gruezi!" with the same "Gruezi!" To the Italian employees I saluted "Buon giorno!" They returned "Buon giorno!" with a smile. I talked with Professor Yasargil in English and German. He was unhappy at the beginning because I brought a recommendation letter from Professor Decker to Professor Krayenbuhl, but he became friendly as we conversed daily. I felt honored when he invited me to his home for dinner. One Saturday in February, Dr. Yonekawa and I drove to his home on a hill overlooking Lake Zurich. We walked over the snow from the gate to the entrance of his house. As soon as I entered his house I was impressed by the many paintings and sculptures. It was a small art gallery. Contrary to my expectation, there were only three guests invited. The other guest was a doctor from the United States. Mrs. Yasargil was a beautiful hostess. The couple told us about their experience in Japan. Professor Yasargil, who was born in Turkey, insisted that the Ainu tribe in Hokkaido had a common origin with the Turkish. I remembered that they had similar faces and thick dark mustaches and hair but could not imagine that Turks could have immigrated to northern Japan. Professor Yasargil was convinced of his theory of Turkish immigration to Japan in ancient times, because he went to Hokkaido to investigate the Ainu tribe. He must have fallen in love with the Ainu people, as with the Japanese in general, because he praised Dr. Kikuchi and Dr. Yonekawa. And then, he held my shoulder and asked me, "Why don't you stay a little longer in Zurich?" He was disappointed when I explained to him the reason why I had to leave Zurich in spring. Yes, I wanted to stay longer, because I liked the life in Zurich.

I was also happy with the life in the Maurers' home. In the bookshelves in my room I found Agatha Christie's *Murder on the Orient Express* and was fascinated by this author, the queen of mystery. I have read one after another of her detective stories. I continued collecting her books even after my return to Japan and now have 65 of her books in my bookshelves. Nevertheless, I had to leave the Maurers, because Christiane arranged another home for the rest of my time in Zurich. She brought me to a big apartment house owned by Mrs. Brunner, a friend of Christiane. She was treasurer of the Zurich Opera House. I did not see Mr. Brunner in her apartment. They seemed separated. I avoided asking Mrs.

Brunner about her husband. My room was in a far end of her apartment and we saw each other seldom except at breakfast. She was a tall woman who carried herself well and dressed well.

An unexpected privilege was granted me. I was not charged if I walked into the opera house with her. It was humiliating to walk along with this tall, well-dressed lady, much taller than I, but it saved me the cost of enjoying opera.

Once in the opera house, no more problem. As soon as the seats are taken, the whole opera house becomes quiet and the overture begins. Spotlights illuminate the curtain, which slowly opens, and the first scene attracts the eyes of everyone in the audience who listens to the brilliant orchestra and passionate singing of soprano and baritone singers. They become excited and then cry at the changing fates of the heroes and heroines. Thus I visited the city opera house often without charge, and enjoyed "Tosca," "Aida," and other operas. It was a special privilege.

March came with warmer weather which melted the snow on the streets. My heart was lifted as the time of my return to Nagasaki approached. It was in the middle of March when Christiane told me about her plan of showing me Gunsbach, the home town of her grandfather, Dr. Schweitzer. I was to leave Zurich alone on a train. As soon as Madelaine Brunner heard the plan, she told me, "I'll accompany you till Basel. We should see Paska together." I agreed, although I did not know what Paska meant and we left Zurich on a train early in the morning of a Sunday.

The town of Basel was dark and quiet when we arrived there after an hour's ride. Shadowy figures of people increased along the roadside. They seemed to expect something to happen. We joined them and pricked up our ears.

First came the dim sound of a flute from a distance. The sound increased its volume in a repeating rhythm. Through the mist appeared a marching group of young men wearing triangular hats and colorful uniforms, with flutes to their lips. I had an illusion of being in a medieval world, because the colorful costumes with tight pants belonged to ancient times. No human voice but only the rhythmic sound of flutes filled the air of Basel. Different groups with different clothes followed the first group. It was an enchanting dream world. I watched the silently passing lines of children in beautiful costumes and women with feather hats. It was an endless march, as if it were engulfing all the town with medieval costumes. One peculiarity was its strange silence. The sound of the flutes spread to all corners of the town but no one spoke a word. Songs were sung, but soon they were buried in the sound of flutes. The audience was completely silent. No shouts of praise or laughter were heard. It was a solemn festival, completely different from the noisy festivals in Japan.

It was a festival, nevertheless. It was the traditional religious festival of Easter repeated for generations in Basel since the Middle Ages. I thanked Madelaine for her kindness in showing me this unique Paska in Basel, and left her at Basel Station to travel to Colmar alone.

After running for one hour along the Rhine the train arrived at Colmar, France. Christiane was waiting for me at the station. Colmar is a small town with a population of 50,000. The name is unfamiliar to the Japanese, but its medieval buildings, including Saint Martin Cathedral, are famous in Europe. The former residence of Bartholdi, who designed the Statue of Liberty in New York, is now the museum of the city. Christiane took me to the museum to show me the famous altar paintings of Grunewald.

From Colmar we rode on a small, local train. Soon the train stopped at a small station. It was Gunsbach, a small village with a few small houses. The biggest building I found in the village was a small church. Two or three hundred meters from the church stood a two-story building on the other side of the road. It was Maison Albert Schweitzer, a memorial museum to Dr. Schweitzer built by Schweitzer himself in 1928. He went to the grammar school in the village. Later he studied theology and medicine in Strasbourg, not very far from this village. He loved this home, and stayed in this house whenever he came to Europe from Lambarene, Africa, for lectures, organ recitals, and for collecting funds for the hospital to serve his black brothers. In this house he wrote many books including *Between the Sea and the Jungle*, *Out of my Life and Thought* and *Philosophy of Life*. His books influenced me. His books motivated me to become a physician. And now I am in this sacred house with his beloved granddaughter, Christiane. I was overwhelmed by emotion.

The Maison was organized and maintained by Miss Ali Silver, his former faithful secretary, who welcomed us with a smile and warm handshake. She took us inside and showed me all the exhibits in the house. There were the writings of Dr. Schweitzer in his grammar school days, and the records evaluating his school work. I was amused to find the cradle in which baby Albert slept. His old organ, music scores, manuscripts and first editions of his own books, and translated books in many languages were exhibited in good order along with many albums and photographs. A big frame on the wall of the last room caught my eye. There was written on the paper a Japanese phrase in large calligraphic letters, "God is Love," with the signature of Kanzo Uchimura, a great Japanese Christian leader.

When I sat alone in Dr. Schweitzer's small bedroom on that evening, looking at the tower of the church through the window framed with ivy leaves, I said to myself, "God is Love,"

# PART III

# 25

# NAGASAKI ROSAI HOSPITAL

In December, 1973, seven months after I had returned from Europe, Professor Sato, the Dean of the Medical School, asked me, "What would you like to do from now on? Do you mind working in Rosai Hospital?"

He had good reason to ask me. While I was in Europe, the new Department of Neurosurgery was officially opened in our medical school on New Year's Day. I had studied neuroradiology in Munich under Professor Decker for three months, had studied microsurgery in Zurich under Professsor Yasargil for three more months, and had come back to Japan via Canada, staying one week in London, Ontario, to see the advanced technique of Professor Charles D. Drake to deal with aneurysm in the deep posterior portion of the brain. What awaited me was the post of Associate Professor in the new department. I had to work under the new Professor Kazuo Mori, a newcomer to Nagasaki, who was more than ten years younger than I. I felt somewhat humiliated. Professor Mori must have been embarrassed to have an older, popular neurosurgeon on his staff. He was polite to me, but I knew that he did not need me. I knew also that my presence was an obstacle for younger neurosurgeons who wanted to be promoted, but I did not know where I should go. Often came to my mind the casual words of Professor Yasargil in Zurich: "Microsurgery of the brain arteries puts pressure on your heart. One should not keep on doing this kind of surgery. Fifty-five years of age should be the age limit for microsurgery." Within a month, on the fourth of January, I was to reach the age of 55 years. I would have worked in the University Hospital for 19 years and eleven months by my next birthday. This might be the right time to resign from my alma mater. I answered Professor Sato,"Yes, I'll resign at the end of this year."

The Nagasaki Rosai Hospital is in Sasebo, not very far from Nagasaki. The Director of the hospital at that time was Professor Emeritus Saburo Nagai, who had retired from Nagasaki University after a stroke which had left him partly paralysed with a speech impediment. He was admitted to the University Hospital this winter because he caught cold and developed pneumonia. He became critical once in December. Dean Professor Sato might have considered me as a successor to Professor Nagai in case he succumbed to the illness. He had sympathized with me when I failed to become the professor of neurosurgery in spite of my long devotion to neurosurgey.

Miwa had no objection to my new assignment. She knew only too well my situation in the medical school. Thus I started to work at the Nagasaki Rosai Hospital on my 55th birthday.

I had known Professor Nagai since he came to Nagasaki as the Professor of Orthopedics. I had helped him in an international symposium of orthopedic surgery held in Unzen National Park. Therefore I was glad to work as a neurosurgeon under his supervision. Besides, I knew well Dr. Shimada, the Assistant Director, who was a surgeon interested in neurosurgery. Once a week I used to see neurosurgical cases at the out-patient clinic, and sometimes I operated on patients with the assistance of Dr. Shimada. All the staff knew me, because they were graduates of Nagasaki University School of Medicine. I was not a stranger in the Rosai Hospital.

One of the apartment houses for doctors was provided for me. I moved to this apartment, leaving Miwa in Nagasaki. Twice a week I drove to Nagasaki. On Wednesday I visited the University Hospital, and on Saturday I went home directly from the Rosai Hospital. It took about one and a half hours to drive from Sasebo to Nagasaki, but the course through the Saikai Bridge crossing the neck of Omura Bay was a scenic driveway called the "Pearl Line" running along the beautiful bay surrounded by the green of nature. The view was dramatic in the evening when the sun set and the moon came out from the shoulder of a mountain. Often I stopped my car to watch the serene beauty of a "Pearl Bay" evening.

It was early morning when I left Nagasaki. In winter it was still dark. Gradually the sky becomes brighter. Suddenly the sun rises from the eastern mountain and the rippling waves shine over

"Pearl Bay." It is a familiar scene in old Japanese paintings. One never gets tired of looking at the scene. In spring, the cherry flower buds enlarge until they suddenly burst into bloom and decorate the lakeside intermittently, as if to welcome my car with an arch of cherry blossoms.

By spring Dr. Nagai had recovered from his severe illness, and had returned to his work as the Director of the Rosai Hospital. It was not easy to understand his words because of his speech impediment. We hesitated to ask him more than twice, and tried not to approach him. As a result he had to stay alone in his office, interrupted only by the visit of his Assistant Director, who had to consult with him often. I felt sorry for Dr. Nagai, and tried to visit him once in a while, even though I spoke to him much more than he did to me.

There was a big rehabilitation department in the Rosai Hospital, because "Rosai" is a Japanese abbreviation of "occupational injury" and many orthopedic patients were in this hospital. No other hospital in Sasebo had such a large rehabilitation unit. One of the reasons I was attracted to this hospital was its good rehabilitation facilities. The setting was too good to be used solely for orthopedic patients. It should be used for neurological patients as well. I dreamed of building a center of neurosurgery in Sasebo, and this was an ideal hospital for the purpose. The location of the Rosai Hospital is in a suburb of Sasebo, but it can be reached from other communities through its good transportation system. A neurosurgical emergency center in this hospital would solve the problem of medical emergencies in Sasebo and its suburban communities.

Dr. Shimada had been trained for a period in neurosurgery at the Tokyo Rosai Hospital, and two surgeons in this hospital had experience helping me with neurosurgical operations in the University Hospital. They could handle head injuries. They would help me organize a department of neurosurgery in this hospital, where young neurosurgeons in Nagasaki University could find posts in the future. This projected neurosurgical center became my dream in the Rosai Hospital.

I explained this plan to Professor Mori, and asked his guarantee to send his staff members when I needed them. I asked Dr. Nagai to arrange purchase of a computerized tomographic (CT) scanner for the hospital. A neurosurgical intern was assigned one year later, but the expensive new machine was not purchased because of its high cost, 250 million yen at that time.

Five years earlier, in 1968, on my way from Loma Linda, I had stopped at Rochester, Minnesota, to visit the Mayo Clinic. I met there a Japanese woman, a graduate of Tsuda College, who was studying speech therapy. After coming to Sasebo, I happened to remember that she had come back to Japan and was working in an institute in Tokyo as a specialist in speech therapy. A good idea came to my mind: I should invite her to Sasebo to participate in a seminar on speech therapy. Dr. Nagai approved my plan, because he himself was suffering from speech disability. After consulting with Miss Hiroko Nakashima, our speech therapist, I wrote a letter to Miss Asanuma. To our delight she consented.

Responding to the invitation letter from Dr. Kondo, the chief of the Rehabilitation Division, and Miss Nakashima, many people came to the hospital to attend the seminar on "Speech Therapy of Dysphasia." Not only the rehabilitation workers but also specialists in psychiatry and otology came to listen to Miss Asanuma's two-hour lecture on "Fundamentals of Speech Dysfunction and its Treatment" and to participate in the hot discussions which followed. The lecture was appreciated by all and the project was a success.

This was a good opportunity for the Department of Oto-rhinolaryngology of the medical school, too. Another lecture was given at the University Hospital with a big audience of various specialties. Throughout these seminars I learned more about Miss Asanuma. She had been an invalid child, and had stayed at home without going to school, but she had kept studying hard at home until she passed the entrance examination to Tsuda College. She had missed opportunities to be married. Poor health was one of the reasons.

In Sasebo she stayed in our apartment house, and Miwa took care of her. The three of us visited famous azalea gardens in Takeo and Omura, because it was the best season for azaleas in Kyushu. She enjoyed the whole tour and went back to her headquarters in the Senility Research Institute founded by the Tokyo Metropolitan Government.

Ten years had passed since Dr. Albert Schweitzer died in Lambarene. The year 1975 was also a centennial anniversary of the birth of Dr. Schweitzer. Many memorial events were planned all over the world. The Nagasaki Branch of Schweitzer's Friends Society also wanted to have a memorial meeting in Nagasaki. I consulted with Dr. Koyano, the local leader of the Society, and with Dr. Minoru Nomura in Tokyo, who had worked with Dr. Schweitzer in Lambarene for some time, and planned a memorial concert with Christiane and the Nagasaki Symphony Orchestra. The orchestra members were delighted with the plan, and Mr. Yasunaga, the conductor of the Kyushu Symphony Orchestra, agreed to conduct again,and promised the help of the Kyushu Orchestra members. Christiane was more than happy to have another chance to play in Nagasaki, and selected Mozart's popular piano concerto No. 26 in D Major, K537, known as "Coronation." The new Concert Hall of Nagasaki City was reserved for the concert. I had to design the program again and sell the tickets.

I remembered a photograph of Dr. Schweitzer which I saw in a room of the First Department of Medicine. It was taken at the time of his Nobel Prize Award speech at Oslo in 1954 when he was 79 years old. He held both hands in front of him as if he were thanking the audience for their applause. His happy smile reflects his warm personality as a philosopher of "Reverence for Life" and a humanitarian who practised "Brotherhood of All Human Beings." His deep furrows are the record of his long life devoted to his African patients. It was a magnificent picture bringing us closer to this great man, who died ten years ago. I went to Professor Takaoka, and asked his permission to use this photograph in the poster of our memorial concert. He permitted the use, and a large poster was designed to include the photo and a caption in Japanese calligraphy heralding "A Memorial Concert for Dr. Albert Schweitzer to celebrate the 100th anniversary of his birth."

The photograph of Dr. A. Schweitzer was also printed on the front page of the program, which listed the music to be played and the names of the performers. An introduction by Dr. Nomura of Schweitzer's Friends Society, and comments on the music by Dr. Nakamura were added on the following pages. The next problem was how to sell the tickets. The "*Usagi-kai*" helped me a great deal with this problem.

The "*Usagi-kai*" was founded by Mrs. Sagan, the wife of Dr. L. A. Sagan who came to Nagasaki in 1960 as a staff member of the Atomic Bomb Casualty Committee and was investigating the effects of the atomic bomb on the survivors. Ginetta Sagan was born in Italy. She had had the sad experience of losing her parents during the war. After I took her to an orphanage called "Koyo-ryou," she became a sponsor of orphanages in Nagasaki which were filled with "war orphans." Her energetic activity to help orphans impressed her Japanese friends and students and they formed "*Usagi-kai* " (Rabbits Club), a volunteer group to help the orphans.I became one of the members and acted as an executive manager and an interpreter for Ginetta. The previous concert in 1972 was a charity concert to raise funds for "*Usagi-kai.*" This time again, "*Usagi-kai*" helped me with the Nagasaki Branch of the Schweitzer's Friends Society and Nagasaki Nepal Society. More than three hundred members of "*Usagi- kai*" worked to sell the tickets.

Christiane came to Nagasaki on October 3 with her fiance, Steve Engel. She soon started rehearsal with the Nagasaki Symphony Orchestra. As the day of the concert approached, she became nervous, but Steve soothed her nerves with good jokes. He was a short man with a dark beard. He found many troubles in our old house and fixed them all with his skill and humming. Christiane seemed to trust him very much.

The concert on October 13 was a success. Mozart's piano concerto, "Coronation," was played after the speech by Dr. Minoru Nomura on "The Life and Work of Dr. Albert Schweitzer." The performance of Christiane and the Nagasaki Symphony Orchestra was better than the last one. I had memorized the beautiful melodies during repeated rehearsals and they echoed in my ears long after the concert. Christiane was satisfied with the good concert and went back to Steve's house in California. They were married in Gunsbach the next spring. Christiane Eckert gained a new family name of Engel, which means "angel" in German.

Dr. Nagai, the Director of the Rosai Hospital, gave up seeing patients in the clinic, because the patients could not understand his poorly pronounced words, but he had no intention of giving up his position as the head of the hospital. He suspected that I had sneaked into the hospital to take his position, and was determined to protect his post. No new stroke attacked him and he looked healthy except for his hemiparesis. I was neither a superintendent nor his assistant, but was given a strange title of a Medical Consultant in my second year in the Rosai Hospital. It sounded like a special title, but no new work was added to my clinical work of neurosurgery. I wanted a Computerized Tomographic Scanner rather than a title, but there seemed no possibility of buying this expensive x-ray machine.

It was in April, 1976, more than two years after I moved to the Rosai Hospital, that Professor Yasukuni Tsuji called me to his office in the University Hospital. He started bluntly, "Could you go to the Yahata Hospital in Kita-kyushu? Please, go there and work as the Director for the sake of Nagasaki Unversity."

I could not resist his words "for the sake of Nagasaki University," and I answered, "Yes, I will, if it's good for our school, but give me time to talk with my wife."

I expected objections from Miwa, because we would have to move to Kita-kyushu, four hours journey from Nagasaki where we have our house. However, she did not oppose my new assignment. "I'll follow you wherever you go, if you think you must go."

I called Professor Tsuji on the telephone, and told him Miwa's consent. He was glad and thanked me.

It was against custom in our medical school that Professor Tsuji, who belonged to the First Department of Surgery, asked me, who belonged to the Second Department of Surgery, to take a post in a hospital affiliated with the First Department. There had been rivalry between the First Department and the Second Department of Surgery as between the First and the Second Department of Medicine. Any vacant post of one department must be filled by a doctor belonging to the same department. It was exceptional in my case. Professor Tsuji and I were graduated from the Saga High School in the same year. Dr. Hatano, my former classmate at the medical school, belonged to the First Department of Surgery until he was promoted to Professor of Anesthesiology. We were good friends, and met and talked often. My good relationship with the First Department of Surgery was often criticized by the staff of the Second Department of Surgery. Some of them dared to ask me cynically, "Which Department do you belong to?" Therefore, this offer of the post of the Director of a city hospital from the First Department surprised me and other people.

Soon I learned the reason for this unprecedented appointment. Several surgeons in the First Department of Surgery were asked to take the post of the present director, who wanted to retire. No one accepted the offer. The Yahata City Hospital was the smallest of the six city hospitals in the city of Kita-kyushu. It occupied an old building built shortly after the war. The hospital did not function well, and was constantly in debt, with only one hundred out-patients per day for the 250 bed hospital. The city wanted to close the hospital or rebuild it as the badly-needed emergency medical center of the city. An emergency medical center is difficult for any medical director to supervise. Another problem was the powerful labor union in this hospital. There was not a single union but two unions belonging to two different political parties. No wonder that every candidate turned down the offer of the directorship of this hospital. Finally Professor Tsuji mentioned my name as the last candidate. To his amazement all the staff of the Yahata Hospital as well as the staff of the First Department of Surgery at Nagasaki University consented to my appointment.

I asked Professor Tsuji to postpone my appointment, because our son was to be married at the end of April. The present Director, Dr. Watanaba, agreed to stay in his post until August, although he intended to retire in April because of his asthmatic bronchitis. Toshio, our son, was married on April 29 at the age of twenty-eight, as I was married to Miwa on the same day at the same age in 1946. The wedding was conducted by me in a hotel located close to the monument of the atomic bomb. Our close friends and a few relatives attended the simple wedding and the dinner. It was a good, quiet wedding, although the weather was not good. Toshio and the new bride left for Unzen National Park by car in the rain and storm.

I also wanted to travel with Miwa before we moved to Yahata, Kita-kyushu. She had never had the experience of traveling abroad in her 30 years of married life. She had always stayed at home in Nagasaki while I was abroad for my study four times, five years in total. She worked hard to help my poor financial status and survived the loneliness in my absence. She never complained or grumbled. I planned to take her on an overseas tour as an expression of my appreciation.

We traveled in a tour group organized by Japan Air Lines. Miwa enjoyed a two week tour of Europe, starting from Copenhagen and stopping at London, Paris, Geneva, Rome, and Athens before coming home. Miwa's niece and her family welcomed us in London. In Geneva I visited my old friend, Gilbert Beguin, for the first time since we had parted in Ann Arbor in 1952, and met his wife and a newborn baby. Miwa loved the walk along Lake Geneva and enjoyed the cable car climbing up to the top of Mont Blanc.

The only problem I had after the tour was an onset of severe diarrhea due to a contaminated meal in Bangkok Airport on our way home. I suffered repeated diarrhea and was admitted to the Rosai Hospital. I attended the farewell party planned by the hospital staff, but could not eat anything. Slowly I recovered by the time of the farewell party in Nagasaki arranged by the two departments, the Department of Neurosurgery and the Second Department of Surgery. Professor Tsuji of the First Department of Surgery and two professors of medicine gave me warm messages of farewell. There were also many other professors and associate professors of many departments. I was glad to see so many colleagues of our medical school come together, despite the barriers and rivalries among departments, to congratulate my start as Director of an important public hospital,

I left Nagasaki by car at the end of August but had to leave Miwa in the Saga National Hospital on the way, because Miwa complained of severe abdominal pain. I could not stay with her while she was being examined because I had to be in Kita-kyushu by next morning. Though she soon recovered, her sudden illness seemed an ominous beginning for our life in Yahata.

# 26

# YAHATA HOSPITAL

Not far from Yahata Station stood the Yahata Hospital of the City of Kita-kyushu. It has a small mountain behind the building. One might see a cable car running up and down the slope of the mountain. At the foot of this mountain there is a group of public buildings, including the public library facing the crossing roads. On the other side of the road stands the Yahata Hospital. This hospital was built in 1950 and was called the Yahata City Hospital until the City of Yahata became a district of Kita-kyushu City, which started fifteen years ago as a big new city combining five former cities. Still the old name of Yahata City Hospital is more familiar to the citizens than the new, long name.

If one drives to the west of the hospital, one will find two other hospitals in close proximity. One is the Hospital of the Yahata Steel Company, and another is the Saiseikai Hospital, a public hospital belonging to the Red Cross Society. The Yahata Steel Company had been the oldest and the biggest steel manufacturing center in Japan, but it is no longer as active as it was. Many factories have moved to modern buildings in other cities. The big chimney painted "1901" no longer pollutes the air with smoke. The population of Yahata decreased as the air became cleaner. No wonder that the Yahata Hospital is not as busy as it was years ago.

On my first day in Yahata, I stepped inside the Yahata Hospital. The old wooden floor creaked. The Director's office was dark and narrow. The hospital needed a new building. Dr. Furukawa, the Assistant Director, introduced me to the staff of the hospital, There were only fifteen doctors for twelve divisions. None of them was young. There was no pediatrician, no dermatologist, no ophthalmologist, and no otorhinolaryngologist to fill the vacant posts. Not only the building but also the staff needed a total shake-up. I realized my grave responsibility.

Doctors were seeking reconstruction of the hospital, but they were not happy about the emergency work. However, the rationale for the reconstruction of the hospital was to make this hospital the emergency medical center for the city, with its one million population. In this megalopolis, which started in 1963 as a new city consisting of five old cities, Moji, Kokura, Tobata, Wakamatsu and Yahata, there were 79 hospitals and 879 clinics according to the survey in 1973. But only four of these hospitals accepted emergency cases, whereas seven times more hospitals received emergency cases in Fukuoka, the second largest city in Fukuoka Prefecture after Kita-Kyushu.

The good old days are gone. Physicians no longer want to treat patients at night. Leisure is more attractive than patients to younger doctors. They do not stay in the hospital on Sundays and holidays. Even if they stay at home, they refuse to see patients at night or on Sunday. Employees do not want to work after the regular working hours and request extra payment for extra work. Otherwise, they switch to an easier workplace. Surgeons and physicians hesitate to treat emergency cases of head injury and stroke, because they do not want to be involved in lawsuits, which are rapidly increasing in Japan as well as the United States. As a result, they refuse to treat acute emergency patients at night on the grounds that a neurosurgeon or cardiologist should see these patients. The patients are carried around the city at night in a search for the specialists who are hiding somewhere. The anger and discontent of citizens increased every year, and they blamed the city for not setting up enough emergency clinics. The city asked the medical associations to organize a committee to discuss the problem of medical emergency. At the end of 1974 a municipal emergency clinic was started in the Hospital for Contagious Diseases, accepting patients on Sunday and at night. The medical associations of the five districts opened five subcenters on Sunday and in the evening but closed after midnight. The unsolved problem was to find a hospital for the critically injured or ill patients who needed admission to a hospital for further treatment.

Osaka with eight million population is a much larger megalopolis. The average incidence of medical emergency in Osaka on Sunday was 6,400, and 400 of them needed hospital care. If this rate is applied to the city of Kita-kyushu, 50 of 800 patients would need hospitalization on each Sunday. Actually, the city ambulances alone carried approximately 25 patients on Sunday looking for hospitals to admit them. Negotiation with hospitals by telephone takes a long time and is often in vain. Sometimes it takes more than an hour to find a hospital for admission. The waste of time kills many patients who might be saved if treated sooner. The common apology of doctors is, "I am not a specialist. The patient should be treated by a neurosurgeon." In the hospitals which had a department of neurosurgery, they seldom had vacant beds for emergency cases, and their neurosurgeons were not in the hospital on Sunday. Another excuse was that x-ray and laboratory technicians were not available on Sunday and at night. Year after year the automobile accidents increased and the need for facilities to treat injuries at night and on Sunday increased as well. The anxiety of citizens increased likewise, and they blamed the city and medical professions.

The Committee of Emergency Medicine submitted a recommendation to the city. This proposal in May, 1976 emphasized the urgency of setting up the second-stage and third-stage emergency centers in the city. It said, "The second-stage emergency medical center should be a new hospital or a new unit of a city hospital." "A city hospital" meant the Yahata Hospital. In the chapter on "the third-stage emergency medical center," the National Hospital in Kokura was named as the candidate, because the National College of Industrial Medicine to be built in Yahata was still in the planning stage. However, the National Hospital refused to accept the recommendation on the ground that it had no department of neurosurgery. Without the promise of a third-stage center for a back-up, the building plan of a new Yahata Hospital with the second-stage emergency medical center was approved by the Mayor of Kita-kyushu.

I demanded that the city should add a department of neurosurgery to the Yahata Hospital as a minimum requirement to accept emergency cases of head injury. I requested a change in the construction plan of the hospital building in order to have a neurosurgical unit and x-ray examination rooms equipped not only with conventional x-ray machines but also the latest model CT scanner made in England. The city was reluctant to approve my request to purchase machinery and other equipment for the neurosurgical unit, costing the city more than 500 million yen. I insisted that we could not start an emergency medical center without a department of neurosurgery with the necessary resources and personnel. The Mayor yielded to my plea at last.

It was on December 21, 1976, three months after my appointment as the Director, that the construction of the new Yahata Hospital with a new department of neurosurgery began on the revised blueprint. A ceremony to inaugurate the construction was led by the Mayor, who put a spade into the ground in front of representative citizens of the city.

The loud noise of construction filled the air outside the old hospital for one year and eight months. Bulldozers dug the ground deeper and deeper. Concrete mixers kept working all day. The inpatients were irritated by loud noise from the machines. The doctors had to raise their voices when talking with out-patients. As time passed, we gradually became accustomed to the roar of construction, and our hope of seeing the completed new hospital grew larger. On the other hand, the difficulty of securing the necessary new staff members became increasingly evident.

A large number of employees are needed to operate a 246-bed hospital with forty beds for emergency cases and six beds in the intensive care unit. Negotiation with the city officials on the number of employees to be hired was not easy. The nurses and their labor union demanded a large number of nurses in each department. The technicians and the other labor union requested a good number of personnel for the laboratories.

More difficult was to hire and assign the new medical staff. Doctors of four specialties—physician, surgeon, pediatrician and neurosurgeon—must be ready for emergency cases in the hospital at any time of the day or night. This means four doctors on duty at night. In addition, an obstetrician, an anesthetist, two surgeons and two neurosurgeons must be on call. It requires a large number of doctors. In other hospitals night duty or night call comes only once or twice a month. In the Yahata Hospital, we cannot ask doctors to be on duty too often. A new pediatrician was assigned from Nagasaki University who unequivocally stated, "Twenty-four hour care of sick children is impossible unless we have at least eight pediatricians."

I had a long negotiation with him to cut down the number to six from eight. Ten surgeons, eight internists, six neurosurgeons, six pediatricians, in addition to an obstetrician/gynecologist, a plastic surgeon, an orthopedic surgeon, a urologist, an anesthetist, an ophthalmologist, a dermatologist, a dentist, a pathologist, and a radiologist would make a total of fifty-five staff members, more than twice the legally required number of doctors for a 246-bed hospital. I asked the city to approve the employment of fifty-five doctors as the minimum requirement to operate the new Yahata Hospital as the medical emergency center of the city. The city officials were against my plan. They insisted that a large financial deficit would be inevitable with so many employees. The final, favorable decision was made by the Mayor, however, and the city had to accept his judgment.

The next problem was to find the required number of doctors. Mayor Gohei Tani went to Nagasaki University with me and asked the Dean of the Medical School and other professors to find doctors for the Yahata Hospital. The University responded to our request by promising to send the necessary number of doctors from the departments concerned, because most professors were my old colleagues whom I had known in my twenty years of work in the University Hospital. Two Departments, however, could not provide doctors. They were Ophthalmic and Otorhinolaryngological departments. They did not have enough staff to spare for us. The Pediatric Department promised two or three doctors, but not six, because the city of Nagasaki was to open an emergency medical center which had requested a number of pediatricians to work for the center at night. The professor of pediatrics mentioned the name of Professor Jiro Yamashita of Kurume Medical School as a possible sponsor. I went to Kurume as soon as I was told, and met Professor Yamashita, a gentleman and scholar. He sympathized with my situation and promised his help. I felt as if I had met a Savior in the Inferno.

The doctors in Kita-kyushu were mostly graduates of Kyushu University or Kurume Medical School, two old medical schools in Fukuoka Prefecture. Graduates of Nagasaki University were in the minority. In the five other city hospitals there was only one surgeon who graduated from Nagasaki University. Even in the Yahata Hospital there were not many graduates of Nagasaki. I was the only medical director who belonged to the minority group of doctors in Kita-kyushu. I felt rather isolated at first, but my anxiety disappeared at the first dinner party of directors and assistant directors of all city hospitals.

As soon as I entered the Japanese-style dining room of the New Tagawa Hotel, a doctor approached me and introduced himself as Dr. Eto of the Moji Hospital. He told me that he had been in Saga High School before he entered Kyushu University. We talked about our common friends graduated from Saga High School, including Professor Tsuji who recommended me to the Yahata Hospital. I was surprised to find another graduate of Saga High School, Dr. Tayama of the City Sanatorium. He was much older than I. I had not met him before, but he welcomed me with his friendly smile as a senior graduate from the same high school. The three of us talked about Saga High School with feelings of nostalgia and intimacy.

The Director of the Kokura Hospital, the largest among six city hospitals, was Dr. Toichiro Sawata, a former Professor of Internal Medicine at Kyushu University. He was eighty years old but sat on the seat with his back straight. I went to him and introduced myself. Then I added, "I understand that you were born in Iwate where the famous poet Kenji Miyazawa was also born. I admire him. Particularly I love his last poem: "Never be discouraged by rain."

Dr. Sawata suddenly changed his scholarly rigidity to a friendly smile. "It's good. I was his classmate!" Then he told me about his school life in Morioka Middle School. We toasted together his old classmate and our first meeting. Since that evening he has been friendly to me and helped me in many situations, including the difficult negotiations with the city on the reconstruction of the Yahata Hospital. The Kokura Hospital, also with a reconstruction plan, was an older building than the Yahata Hospital, but the city decided to rebuild the Yahata Hospital first. I felt sorry for Dr.Sawata, but he was not hurt. He simply said, "Our turn will come after your hospital. Never mind."

Actually he was to retire before the Kokura Hospital was rebuilt under the administration of a new director from Kyushu University. He was Professor Emeritus Dr. Yujiro Ikemi, a famous author of books on psychosomatic medicine. When I met him for the first time at a formal dinner, he surprised me. "I heard you know Dr. Akizuki of St. Francisco Hospital."

He knew that I was exposed to the atomic bomb in the University Hospital and he knew about my work for the victims in St. Francisco Hospital, because he was a friend of Dr. Akizuki. He is a Buddhist, but he knew Christianity and studied the Bible, too. We became good friends. And this friendship with the Director of the leading city hospital helped me in many ways, as much as the support from two other Directors who were graduates of Saga High School. They were all graduates of Kyushu University, but it did not matter to me any more. The Director of the Tobata Hospital, Dr. Hisanaga, was not a graduate of Kyushu University, but he was once a resident of the Department of Gynecology at Kyushu University. His grandfather was a pastor and had worked at Doshisha University. We found common topics and he was friendly to me, too. The Director of the Wakamatsu Hospital was a young, amiable person. I found no bitterness but good will and cooperative attitudes in the leaders of the city hospitals in spite of our different medical backgrounds. I am grateful for their support during my difficult time in Kita-kyushu.

Construction of the new Yahata Hospital was finally finished in August, 1978. It cost the city 2.6 billion yen. After all patients moved to the new building, the old building was torn down and removed to make a parking area, a much larger parking area than that of any other city hospital. The orange-colored exterior of the six-story building looked warm and beautiful. Each floor had a veranda, which saved the whole building from monotony. In front of the porch there is a dome-style roof with a round glass window at its top, giving an image of a hotel rather than a hospital. The large hall inside the entrance leads to the spacious waiting room. The color of the wall and the floor is either orange or cream yellow, giving a warm feeling. The nurses' stations are in the center, and the long lines of wards are on both sides of the nurses' station, which is open to the wards and to the elevator. Many wards have oxygen and vacuum suction piped in for seriously ill patients. The Intensive Care Unit has six beds and a monitoring system to show the patients' respiration and heart rates on computer screens. This modern ICU and forty emergency beds helped to get recognition for the Yahata Hospital as the critical emergency center in northern

Kyushu, and an annual subsidy from the government was guaranteed. The new Yahata Hospital became the center of the so-called "Kita-kyushu system" of emergency medicine, which started on October 1, 1978.

We expected some confusion at the beginning of the new system, but it worked smoothly. There was no rush of primary care patients, because the city informed the public about the new system through television and other mass media for one month prior to the start. In the first month, patients with mild illness or injury came sometimes directly to the hospital, and we had to explain to them that our hospital accepts only those cases referred from the primary emergency medical stations. However, such mistakes became rare in the following months. Every night several cases were referred from the primary emergency stations or hospitals, and emergency surgery was often performed until morning.

In addition to doctors of four specialties, four nurses, one pharmacist, one x-ray technician, and one laboratory technician, eleven staff in total, stayed in the hospital every night. Besides, six doctors including surgeons, neurosurgeons and an anesthetist, and two nurses were at home on call for emergency surgery. Such a big team was needed to be ready for the emergency medical work at night and on holidays. I took night duty every week, because there were only four neurosurgeons in the hospital including myself.

The number of outpatients increased steadily after the new hospital started and doubled before long. The large parking area was filled with patients' cars, and another parking place for employees had to be found. Visitors thronged every day to visit the emergency patients who were admitted during the previous night. They saw the beauty and good setup of the new hospital. No wonder the good reputation of the Yahata Hospital spread without advertisement or promotion. The discharged patients told their friends, "I was sent to the Yahata Hospital by an ambulance car at night. The doctors and nurses in the hospital were kind and skilled. I did not realize that there was such a good hospital in Yahata."

Not only the patients but also their friends wanted to be admitted to the Yahata Hospital if they became ill.

I emphasized "human harmony" whenever I was asked to give a talk to our employees. Three factors important in any enterprise are the right time, the right place and good human relationships. It was the right timing of Heaven that the Yahata Hospital was rebuilt with new equipment and new staff to meet the need for emergency medical care in the city. The hospital is also in the right place, in the middle of the large city of Kita-kyushu with easy access from all districts. To top it off "human harmony" is needed: good team work based on smooth human relations. This "human harmony" is the most important key to good hospital care and good treatment for the sick in the neighborhood. To be kind to the patients as if they were our own family or friends, we hospital staff must be a big family and good friends, helping and cooperating with each other. Not only did I impart this principle to our employees, but also I tried to be a good friend to each one of them.

# 27

# THE LIFE LINE

I did not know that Ruth Hetcamp, who came to Kyushu with Maria von Trapp several years ago, was the founder of the "Tokyo Life Line" until I was invited to the organizing committee of the "Kita-kyushu Life Line" in my second year in Kita-kyushu. I wondered why I had been invited to this committee, so I asked Dr. Sohei Akiyama and his wife, the planners of the new Life Line. Mrs. Akiyama's answer was, "Because Miss Ruth Hetcamp recommended you." Then she told me about the activities of the existing Life Lines in Japan. The Life Line is a voluntary organization which tries to prevent suicide by telephone counselling.

According to the article by Dr. Akiyama, the first attempt to prevent suicide by telephone counselling was begun in 1953 by Rev. Chad Valla in London. Life Line spread rapidly to the whole world, including Switzerland, Germany, Australia and the United States. There are now 167 branches in England alone. It was called "Life Line" or "Samaritans" in England, but it has different names in other countries. Regardless of the name, they contribute tremendously to the prevention of suicide by answering the calls of suffering clients.

In 1971 the "Life Line in English" for foreign clients was opened in Tokyo by Miss Ruth Hetcamp, a German missionary, as the first Life Line in Japan. This stimulated Japanese Christians in Tokyo, and they established the "Tokyo Life Line." Then new stations were set up in Osaka and Okinawa. The "Kita-kyushu Life Line" was the fourth in Japan.

I knew none of the organizing committee members until I attended their meeting, but their sympathy for those who have problems and their enthusiasm to prevent suicide impressed me. They welcomed me and soon we became good friends and faithful comrades. There were Protestant ministers, Rev. Tetsu Akiyama and Rev. Eiichi Murakami. There were college professors, Mr. Niimura and Mr. Hotai. There were lawyers, Mr. Iemon Yamaguchi and Mrs. Mitsuyo Sugisaki. There were doctors like me and Dr. Kaizo Amano, a former president of a medical association. The rest were housewives, including capable Mrs. Akiyama and Mrs. Tomiyasu. The big hurdle, as with any similar project, was the problem of funds. Dr. Akiyama proposed asking for financial help from the Asahi Welfare Foundation, which built the Kokura Memorial Hospital. I objected.

"If our organization is supported by a newspaper company like Asahi Press, other newspapers will not cooperate with us, and the citizens will think that our project is the Asahi Newspaper's project. We must be independent. We should all share the responsibility of financing this project. We can ask the public for donations only after contributing whatever we ourselves can offer. I promise to donate in my capacity."

Other members agreed and promised their donations. The fund was not yet sufficient, and Dr. Akiyama and others visited their friends and asked for their donations. On the basis of this precious fund the "Kita-kyushu Life Line" was founded on July 25, 1977. Miss Ruth Hetcamp came from Tokyo and gave us a congratulatory speech with her familiar smile at the inauguration party held in the Kita-kyushu Center of Consultation on the Problems of Youth.

Our telephone counselling actually started on August 15, the date on which Japan had surrendered 32 years ago. Fifty-two volunteer counsellors had been trained ahead of time. They worked in turn from 5:00 to 9:00 p.m., answering calls and giving advice on the telephone. Later, after the second and third training courses, many new volunteers were added, and the time of counselling was extended: from 1:00 to 9:00 p.m. by the following April, from 10:00 a.m. to 9:00 p.m. in January, 1979, and from 9:00 a.m. to midnight in 1981. At last for 24 hours every day, since October 1, 1982. The number of telephone calls also increased year after year. It was 961 in the first year, and 11,159 in 1981, an increase of more than ten times in five years. In the five years, suicide wish was confessed by 1,343 callers, 519 men and 824 women. The "Kita-kyushu Life Line" saved many people from suicide. Although the Life Line's activity was not publicized, its contribution to the community should be recognized.

The principle of counselling is "to listen and to understand," as Professor Niimura, a psychologist, and Dr. Akiyama, a psychiatrist, emphasized frequently. Preaching and giving advice too soon would not make good counselling. You must sit patiently and listen carefully to what clients tell you. This attitude of acceptance will give support and encouragement to the discouraged and despairing clients. They can review their problems and see themselves with the eyes of others, admitting their own faults and mistakes. The solution can be found by the clients themselves during the process of the conversation on the telephone, even if they reject orders and advice from others. An aggressive person cannot be a good counsellor. The secret of good education as well as the secret of success in business might lie in this human psychology. It is the same in conferences. After giving the chance to express opinions to everyone, the chairman can give his conclusion as the consensus of the group. "A good leader is a good listener."

Marriage problems, relations with the opposite sex, and incompatibility account for more than half of the calls for telephone counselling. Whenever there were difficult questions about illness and sex, the counsellors suggested that the clients call me and ask my advice. I had to answer their questions on the telephone when they called me.

I was asked to give a lecture on sex counselling in the training course for volunteer counsellors. The problem of sex is not limited to the field of obstetrics or gynccology. It is also a mental and cultural problem, as I wrote in my guide book on sex counselling, *From Eros to Agape*.

"Sex is a part of human nature inseparable from the human life in a society. It must be understood and evaluated properly. It is a mistake to despise it or ignore it, as it is also wrong to overestimate it. It is not enough to learn the biological development of sex and anatomy and the physiology of sex in human beings. We must extend our knowledge and understanding to the social, ethical and legal aspects of sex in a given society, in addition to religious restrictions and bias on sex. A fair constructive counselling is possible only on the grounds of this knowledge and understanding.

We must avoid prejudiced personal judgement based on our limited personal experience and bias."

As a neurosurgeon I know the location of the sex center in the hypothalamus of the brain. I have also observed the delayed growth of sex organs due to a tumor in the hypothalamus, amenorrhea caused by a pituitary tumor, and precocius puberty accelerated by pinealoma. Abnormal hyper- or hypo-secretion of hormone is sometimes caused by hydrocephalus involving compression of the hypothalamus with dilated third ventricle. The hypothalamus is also the center of emotion. And emotional changes influence hormonal secretion and sexual behaviour. The sexual drive must be controlled by the frontal lobe of the brain, the center of intelligence and integrity. All past experience is stored in the temporal lobe, the human computer. The brain and sex are closely related in a mysterious way. There are delicate aspects of sex only neurosurgeons or neurophysiologists can understand. In my guide book *From Eros to Agape*, I wanted to emphasize the moral and spiritual aspects of sex which had been neglected in other books on sex education. In the last chapter I concluded:

"More important than sex education is education about humanity. The training to make a responsible, independent adult who treats other human beings with respect, care and politeness, will prevent irresponsible sexual behaviour and prepare a human being to become a good parent for the child to be born. If the parents love each other and work together to build a good happy home, their children will love them and want to become a good father and mother like their parents. They develop good habits and learn self-control, without being misled by the blind sex drive.

"A man and a woman seek each other and want to be married to share the joy of sexual contact. When a baby comes as the result, they feel responsibility and a new kind of love. It is no longer naive, selfish love or affection, but unselfish love which one enjoys giving and for which one is willing to sacrifice oneself for the happiness of others. This is no longer 'eros,' sexual love, but parental love of devotion and sacrifice, a reflection of the holy love, agape of God.

"This unselfish love sacrifices everything for the growth and happiness of the child and protects the child with warmth and devotion. It is similar to the agape of God. It is directed to the parents' own child alone at first, but it would extend gradually to other children, to all young people, to all neighbors and all citizens. It should be elevated to compassion for strangers, foreigners, outsiders, sinners and enemies, as Jesus Christ ordered us and proved himself in his short life culminating in his sacrifice on the cross."

The 50 hours of training in four months for volunteer counsellors were repeated every year thirteen times, and there are now more than 180 active counsellors working in turn for the 24-hour service of the "Kita-kyushu Life Line." In the last decade many new Life Lines were born in Japan. Twenty-seven Life Lines were registered by the end of 1986, and the "Kita-kyushu Life Line" is one of the most active Life Lines in Japan. Therefore the 11th Symposium of Suicide Prevention in Japan was held in Kita-kyushu in 1986.

Besides introducing me to Ruth Hetcamp, who in turn got me a volunteer job with the Life Line, Maria von Trapp in a roundabout way got me another job as well. During our tour of Kyushu I told Maria casually, "The Japanese translation of your books contained improper Christian terminology because they were translated by non-Christian Japanese. I would help you if you need a Japanese translator for your next book." Maria remembered my words. The Tokyo Central Press surprised me one day by asking me to translate Maria's new book, for the reason that "the author asked us to appoint you as the translator."

The title of her new book was, *When the King was Carpenter*. It was a story of the life of Jesus in Nazareth until he left the village. The introduction was interesting. The idea of the book started when her four-year-old daughter asked her, "What did Jesus eat at breakfast?" Maria did not know the answer. She looked for information about the daily home life in Israel at the time of Christ. The information she collected interested her and she decided to write a book on the life of Jesus at his home in Nazareth. This introduction led me to the following chapters and I was fascinated by the whole story. I translated the book into Japanese in three short months. It was fun rather than a labor to translate every word into Japanese.

The Japanese edition of this book came out in September, 1978 with the same picture as the original edition of young Jesus on the cover and the photograph of Maria on the back. My translation received a good review. The book was recommended by the Japanese Library Association as one of the best books for every library. It was not sold in Japan as widely as in the United States, because Christianity is not popular in Japan. Christians make up less than one percent of Japanese population.

It was my first translation and my friends wanted to congratulate me on the publication of this book. One evening in the Nagasaki Catholic Center, 42 persons gathered for celebration. Dr. and Mrs. Akiyama and Mrs. Tomiyasu came from Kita-kyushu in spite of stormy weather. One half of those present were Protestants and another half were Catholic friends. The equal number accurately reflected my friendship with a roughly equal number of Protestants and Catholics in Nagasaki. It also reflected the nature of this new book. The author is a Catholic, as the publisher is, but the translator is a Protestant. It was interesting and it pleased me, because I dislike fanaticism and prejudice. Tolerance of other faiths and beliefs is a key to mutual understanding. It might be the influence of Dr. Albert Schweitzer and Dr. Karl Hilty that had led me to look to the ecumenical movement to help overcome the discords and divisions separating sects and denominations. I was attracted and impressed by the writings of "Mukyokai," or non-church Christians, such as Kanzo Uchimura and Toraji Tsukamoto. I am a non-denominational Christian myself, and I have regular Bible meetings in my home. I am a consultant to a Catholic nunnery and a friend of Protestant ministers.

Near the end of the party, the Rev. Mother of the Franciscan Convent stood on the stage and told the people, "I met Dr. Kawano forty years ago when he was a medical student. I see that he has not changed a bit in the meantime."

It was a happy unforgettable evening to look back on times past and to renew my friendship with old acquaintances of prewar and postwar days. The book by Maria von Trapp triggered this reunion.

# 28

# LUNG CANCER

In the summer of 1977, when reconstruction of the Yahata Hospital was at its peak, my brother in Sasebo called me on the telephone. He said, "The swelling in my jaw has not healed long after having a decayed tooth pulled out, and the dentist suggested that I should visit the University Hospital. Would you make contact with a dentist in the University?"

I called the University Hospital and asked a dentist to examine my brother. A few days later, I went to Nagasaki and saw the x-ray film of my brother's jaw. There was large destruction of the bone. It was a bone metastasis of cancer, as I suspected. The dentist agreed. The common source of metastatic cancer is the lung. I asked the dentist to refer my brother to the Second Department of Internal Medicine.

As we suspected, a small lesion was found in the lung. It is surprising that such a small lesion could make a metastatic lesion in a remote bone, but I know how frequent the bone metastasis of lung cancer is. Not infrequently I found such a metastasis instead of a benign brain tumor after opening a skull. I discovered the original lesion of cancer in the lung only by careful review of the lung x-ray film, or at the autopsy of the lung. Lung cancer often makes metastases, as was also the case with my niece who died nine years earlier, in 1968.

Keiko was the only daughter of my brother in Sasebo. She was my first niece. She was a new discovery for me, who had six brothers but no sister. Our age difference was not much, because her father was the second son of my father and I was the seventh. She was my younger sister rather than a niece as far as her age was concerned.

We lived together when I stayed with my brother's family in my first year of medical school. The family moved to Saga before the end of the war, and then moved again to Sasebo. She had been away from me for nearly twenty years when my brother phoned me from Sasebo.

"Keiko has been in hospital because of her lung disease. Recently she complains of constant severe pain in the lower half of her body. The pain is so severe that she requests injection of narcotics. She cries aloud every night, complaining of pain until the injection is repeated. Her doctor insists that she should be treated in the University Hospital. Please make an appointment for her."

I hurried to Sasebo on the following day and met her doctor in a public hospital. He said, "I thought she had miliary tuberculosis of the lung, but I was wrong." He showed me an x-ray film of Keiko's lung. Small, irregular dots were found in all areas of her lung. At her age of thirty, tuberculosis has a higher probability than cancer, but the dots were too irregular to be miliary tuberculosis. The doctor produced another film, saying, "I took this picture of her spine, because she complained of constant pain in the lower half of the body." The radiograph showed destruction of the vertebrae in the lumbar spine. Pain in the hip and the legs was caused by this destruction of the bone. The nerve branches of the spinal cord were obviously compressed by this metastatic destruction of the spine.

Keiko, lying in bed, looked quite different from what I remembered. Her rich, rosy cheeks were no longer there. Her face was thin and pale. She tried to smile, but she distorted her face in pain. I tried to comfort her. "You'll be all right as soon as we move you to the University Hospital." She nodded to me with obvious delight.

We neurosurgeons have a weapon called chordotomy for intractable pain. It is an operation to interrupt pain sensation in the spinal cord. Chordotomy involves cutting the pain tract, the ascending anterolateral tract in the spinal cord which conveys every pain in the lower body. After this surgery, no pain signals from below the pain tract incision reach the brain. If the tract is cut on the right side, the right lower body is numbed. If it is cut on the left side, pain in the left lower body disappears. I had to cut the tract on both sides of the spinal cord for Keiko. It is not an easy surgery, because along the pain tract runs the motor tract to convey orders from the brain to the muscles in the extremities. If the surgical knife slips and this motor tract were injured, the lower parts of the body would be paralyzed. If the pain tracts were cut insufficiently, pain would remain. It is a delicate and difficult operation.

As soon as Keiko was moved to the University Hospital, all necessary examinations and preparations were made for surgery on the next day. On the morning of the next day, I explained to Keiko about the surgery in an optimistic tone. She nodded at my words. She was then carried to the surgery room, and general anesthesia was started.

Seeing that Keiko was completely unconscious, the anesthetist gave a signal. We turned Keiko from the supine position to the face-down position. After disinfection and draping of the skin along the spine, I pointed the scalpel toward her skin. At the moment someone shouted, "The heart stopped. I cannot hear the heart sound!"

Immediately Dr. Yutaka Goto, Associate Professor of Anesthesiology, gave an order to turn Keiko to the lying position, and started resuscitation using cardiac massage and injection of drugs. After several tense minutes, Keiko's heart started to pulsate again. "What will you do, Dr. Kawano? Do you dare to operate on her?" He asked me and I answered, "Let me do the operation. I'll take all responsibility if anything goes wrong."

Surgery was started again, because I knew she would suffer pain unless I cut her pain tracts. In my mind I shouted, "Forgive me, Keiko." The skin on the spine was incised and opened, disclosing the spinal bone which was partially removed to expose the dura and the underlying spinal cord in the spinal canal. The cord was distorted to make visible the pain tract running along the anterolateral side of the cord. After cutting 4.5mm width of the pain tract on one side, I exposed the other side of the cord at a different level of the spinal cord. Finally I completed bilateral cutting of the anterolateral tracts without causing any damage to the motor tracts running down behind the pain tracts.

The surgery was successful. The pain had disappeared when Keiko woke up from anesthesia in the recovery room. She thanked me with her weak smile. The pain had gone, but she died one month later at the age of thirty years. She had already been worn out from her lung cancer by the time of the chordotomy.

Keiko was an exceptionally young case for lung cancer. I should have known at her death that she invited this unfortunate end as the result of her daily smoking since her days in high school. I did not have enough knowledge about the dangers of smoking until her father became another victim of smoking nine years later.

His cancer in the lung was not diagnosed until a bone metastasis was found in his jaw by a dentist. It was too late to operate on the lung because metastases were already spread outside the lung. My brother was transferred to the Sasebo City Hospital, where his ulcerated stomach had been resected six years ago. I thought he had quit smoking since the operation, but he had not. I was surprised to find him smoking at home a few years after his gastrectomy. Instead of telling him directly, I told my sister-in-law, "Please, stop his smoking. Otherwise, he will develop some other disease." Her answer disappointed me. She said, "After retirement, he has not had much fun in his life. Don't take smoking away from him, for he enjoys smoking."

I said no more. After all, it was none of my business. Now, however, I regret that I did not stop his smoking. People mention heredity, because lung cancer caught him within ten years after it killed his daughter. It was neither heredity nor coincidence. My parents did not die of lung cancer. None of my other brothers died of lung cancer. I started reading articles and information on smoking and illness, and was shocked by many facts which I had not known before.

"At the annual meeting of the Lung Cancer Society in 1966, Nishikawa and his coworker reported on their ten-year study of 3,780 cases of lung cancer in regard to the relationship between lung cancer and smoking. According to them the risk of lung cancer is 10.5 times higher in male and 27.1 times in female heavy smokers than non-smokers" (*Diagnosis and Treatment*, June 1971).

Two years before the death of Keiko, it was already proved that women were more susceptible to lung cancer than men if they smoke. It is surprising that women who smoke have such a high risk of 27 times against 10.5 times of men smokers in Japan. Japanese women must be far more sensitive and delicate than Japanese men. They have less resistance to tobacco than men. Keiko was no exception. It was not by accident that Keiko developed lung cancer and died young, because she was a woman and started smoking in her high school days, either through the influence of her friends or of her father.

According to the survey by Dr. Hammond in the United States, the incidence of lung cancer death among smokers who started smoking before the age of 19 was 5.15 times that of non-smokers, and 14.3 times among smokers who started smoking before age 14. It did not take long before cancer invaded the lung of Keiko, who started smoking in her teens. I discovered another factor, "passive" or "involuntary" smoking! Non-smokers cannot avoid inhaling the harmful smoke if anyone smokes in the same room. And this side-stream smoke is more harmful than the main-stream smoke. It contains much higher concentrations of carcinogens, carbon monoxide, ammonia and other harmful chemical agents. Passive smokers record an elevation of blood pressure, an increase in pulse rate and irritation of the nose and throat. People who have cardiac disease or asthmatic bronchitis suffer aggravated symptoms.

Another report from Aichi Public Health Center tells us that the incidence of asthmatic bronchitis among three-year-old children is ten times higher in homes where mothers smoke than in non-smoking homes. It is possible that the incidence of cancer is higher among children who grow up in smokers' homes. Dr. T. Hirayama surprised the world by his famous report on the higher incidence of lung cancer among wives whose husbands smoke, more than twice that of wives of non-smokers. Another study in Greece confirmed the higher risk of lung cancer among women whose husbands smoke, more than three times that of the controls. Therefore, it was no coincidence or exception that lung cancer killed Keiko, who lived with a smoking father since her birth and started smoking herself in her teenage years.

While I was collecting information on smoking, Mrs. Tomiyasu asked me to speak on health at a high school for a group of mothers, because her two boys were students at the high school. I decided to talk on smoking and health. It was at the beginning of the second semester.

What I told them was: (1) Lung cancer in my brother and his daughter was caused by smoking. (2) There were no symptoms of lung cancer before metastases were found in the bone. (3) The diagnoses of lung cancer were made too late for surgical treatment, as usual in lung cancer. (4) Prevention is far more important than treatment in lung cancer. (5) The best prevention is to avoid smoking and to quit smoking.

The post-war increase of lung cancer deaths in Japan was astonishing, ten times in the first ten years, and 31 times between 1948 and 1982; 33.8 times in males and 26.9 times in females. If more and more young women and students smoke, as they do, the increase in lung cancer will be accelerated. Lung cancer is not the only type of cancer induced by smoking. Smoking will evoke all kinds of cancer, such as cancer of the pharynx, larynx, esophagus, pancreas, liver, uterus and bladder. Stomach cancer is no exception. The higher the number of cigarettes one smokes per day, the higher is the risk of developing stomach cancer. In England many die of chronic bronchitis and emphysema. The rate is five or six times higher among smokers. Everyone knows that World War II and the atomic bomb killed a tremendous number of people in the world, but few know that many more are dying every year because of smoking; more than 350,000 in the United States, 150,000 in Japan, 100,000 in Great Britain and 500,000 in all Europe, two and a half million deaths in the whole world. World War II ended but the smoking epidemic did not come to an end. It is repeated every year, and the victims will increase forever unless we shut out tobacco smoke from this earth. Japan is the worst offender, so far as smoking is concerned. The government has a monopoly of tobacco production and sales. Tobacco is advertised in all kinds of media, not only in magazines, newspapers and billboard, but also on many TV commercials every day. Early in 1900 a law to prohibit smoking of and selling tobacco to people under age twenty was passed in Japan as a good law to protect young people. Nevertheless, cigarette vending machines are standing on many streets in Japan, violating the law by providing cigarettes to anybody regardless of age. No wonder that consumption of cigarettes increases in Japan, while smoking rates are declining in other developed nations, particularly in England, Australia and the United States. Japan is a big nation in the slavery of the tobacco industry.

It is a subject too big for a one hour speech. I finished my talk with the words of Dr. Hirayama: "The best heritage a parent can give to his child is a non-smoking habit. The best guidance a teacher can give to his student is not to smoke."

# 29

# STOCKHOLM

Mrs. Tomiyasu thanked me a few days later. saying, "Your lecture on the other day was impressive. It should be passed on to many others who could not come to our meeting. Would you write it down, please?"

I promised I would. I wrote a manuscript in a hurry and gave it to Mrs. Tomiyasu. The title of the booklet was *Dangerous Tobacco Pollution*. The contents were:

Why do women live longer than men?
Increasing lung cancer
Smoking is the cause of many diseases
Half of heart attacks are due to smoking
One cigarette shortens your life 14 minutes and 30 seconds
Toxicity of nicotine and carbon monoxide
Smoking causes impotence and sterility
Smoking mothers damage their children
Smoking is the biggest source of air pollution
The menace of carbon monoxide hemoglobin
Tobacco pollution has been neglected
The world fighting against tobacco
Japan is a paradise for smokers
Protect the people from tobacco pollution

Every time I visited my brother at the hospital, I noticed gradual deterioration of his physical strength. My sister-in-law was beside my brother and complained to me as she stroked his aching back, "How long will he suffer this pain?"

He had developed carcinomatous pleurisy. The muddy-looking fluid filled the pleural space in spite of repeated removal of the fluid by needle suction.

"Can I use narcotics?"

One day the doctor who was in charge of my brother asked my consent by long-distance telephone. He explained that my brother's severe pain needed narcotics, which might speed up his deterioration. I had to agree. I guessed the end of his life was coming. A few days later I received the news of his death. In the middle of the night, sputum choked him to death. Doctors were too far away to help him. He died only three months after the diagnosis of lung cancer. It was October 31, the very day when Martin Luther listed his 95 items of protest on the door of the Wittenberg Castle Church in 1517.

I felt sorry for him because I was not by his side at the last moment, but my sister-in-law had been with him all the time. I hurried to Sasebo and met her. Contrary to my expectation, she was not crying in despair. Instead, she told me in a tone of relief, "This was good for him. I did not want to see him suffer any longer. His agony has ended. He went to eternal peace, and I am glad for him." It must have been very painful for her to see him suffer.

His funeral was performed in the same Lutheran church where his daughter Keiko had her funeral nine years ago. My brother had been the church organist. Nearly all the church members attended the funeral service. Tears fell from my sister-in-law's eyes as she looked at the coffin in which he was laid with his beloved tennis racket. At the end of the service I stood up in front of a big wreath of flowers given by Mayor Tani of Kita-kyushu City and thanked all who attended the service.

"As a doctor and as a brother of this beloved man I am ashamed that I did not stop his smoking and failed to prevent his lung cancer. I feel deeply sorry for him and his wife, who is left in sorrow. Tobacco killed my niece Keiko, and now it killed my brother. Their deaths should not be wasted. I announce here that I am going to start a war against this dreadful enemy, smoking. Please help me, all of you." One week later my first shot in the battle came with the printing of the aforementioned pamphlet entitled *Dangerous Tobacco Pollution.*

My sister-in-law, who accepted the death of my brother as the end of his pain, felt the loneliness after his death more and more every day. She often told her friends, "I miss him so much that I want to join him soon in Heaven."

One morning in the next Spring, my nephew's wife surprised me on the telephone. My sister-in-law did not come down to breakfast that morning and her daughter-in-law went upstairs to wake her up. She was shocked to find her mother-in-law lying on her bed cold. She called a physician in a hurry, but nothing could be done. She had been dead for hours. I heard the sobbing on the telephone.

The news of her sudden death appalled me. In my confused thought came the memory of a book I had read recently. The title of the book was *The Broken Heart*.. The author was James Lynch, a professor at the University of Maryland. The book was published in 1977, the year my brother died. As soon as I read a review of the book in *Time* magazine, I ordered the book. It came in February and I found it very interesting, good enough for translation into Japanese.

*The Broken Heart* refers to the deep sorrow which can break one's heart. Actually many people have died of a heart attack following deep sorrow. Cardiac arrest due to coronary infarction is reponsible for 55 percent of American deaths, and it occurs in most cases within six months after the death of loved ones.

My sister-in-law also died of a broken heart. Her heart ceased to work under the deep sorrow of missing her dear husband. Only six months after his death, at the peak of the cherry blossom season, she left to join her husband silently in the morning of April 7. She might have felt happy at her departure, expecting to join her beloved one, but it was tragic for her family who were left behind. None of them could be with her to say farewell at her last moment.

At the funeral in the same church where we had her husband's funeral six months earlier, I remembered a famous short poem by Saigyo, a poet monk of the twelfth century,

*I pray I could die under the cherry blossom*
*In the gleam of full moon in the month of full blossom.*

If my brother had not died of lung cancer as a victim of tobacco, my sister-in-law would not have died of a broken heart. In a sense, she was another victim of tobacco. I renewed my determination to fight against tobacco.

Many copies of *Dangerous Tobacco Pollution* were distributed to the high school students and their parents in Kita-kyushu. A number of junior and senior high schools asked me to speak on smoking and health to students. I asked principals to give the booklet to every student. It is difficult to prevent students from smoking unless their parents understand what I teach to children. Some schools made their own copies of my booklet and gave them to students but many more bought our copies.The need increased and we printed again and again, revising the statisical figures accordingly. More than forty thousand copies were distributed within one year. Requests for my speech came from community centers in the city and other institutes, and my booklet was introduced to them, too. But schools were the main customers of my booklets.

A small, intensely loyal group was formed by those who were concerned about the problem of smoking. Mrs. Tomiyasu named the group the "Kyushu Anti-Smoking Society." The main members of this society were Rev. Noboru Arase, Dr. Minoru Tabata of the Health Department of Kita-kyushu City, and Mr. Ryutaro Beppu and Mr. Tadamasa Tsukada, two high school teachers who made an educational movie "In the Smoke of the Cigarette" with the cooperation of their school children. Later Mrs. Shoko Suematsu, a public health nurse, and Mr. Sakae Koga, a children's counsellor of the City, joined us. It was to our advantage that Mayor Tani and Dr. Sakurai, president of the Kita-kyushu Medical Association, were non-smokers and encouraged our movement.

Unbelievable things happened. One year after we started our campaign against smoking, an interesting news item was reported in a local newspaper. The sales of cigarettes in August, 1978 dropped 5.1 percent from the previous year in Kita-kyushu, while the rate was -0.2 percent in the whole of Japan as well as in Fukuoka, the second largest city in Fukuoka Prefecture. The reporter could not understand why. I was excited, because I knew the answer. I remembered what I heard from Mrs. Tomiyasu. In high schools, those students who listened to my speech at the school went home and told their smoker fathers, "Please quit smoking, because I want you to live longer." or, "Don't smoke when we are at home. We have to inhale the side-stream smoke, which might decrease our brain function with its carbon monoxide."

And their fathers either stopped or reduced smoking, to the delight of their mothers. It was a wonderful discovery for me. My yellow booklets were read by the students and brought to their homes, and shown to their parents and other members of the family. As a result the rate of smoking was reduced in Kita-kyushu. Many parents knew of some disadvantages to smoking before, but they found the danger of smoking far beyond their conception. It was easier for smokers to ignore the advice of their wives, but it was harder to resist the pleas of their children. They could no longer smoke inside the house after knowing the effect of side-stream smoke on the intelligence of their children, as emphasized in my booklet. In the long run, teaching children about smoking contributes indirectly to reducing the smoking of their parents and the community they belong to. This new truth was revealed by the newspaper report on the reduction of cigarette sales in Kita-kyushu. It was an unexpected effect of my booklet, which was distributed to more than forty thousand homes in Kita-kyushu.

As soon as I learned of the 4th World Conference on Smoking and Health to be held in Stockholm the following year, I mailed a summary of my paper "Community Education on Smoking through School Children." My application was accepted, and I was given an opportunity to read my paper at the conference.

Reconstruction of the Yahata Hospital was completed, and the management of the new hospital went smoothly. I had nothing to worry about now so I flew to Scandinavia in June, 1979. I was to attend the conference at Stockholm in Sweden and then the Emergency Medical Association Meeting at Oslo, Norway.

In Stockholm, 550 scholars and teachers gathered from 67 countries to discuss the problem of smoking and health. To my amazement, there were only four participants from Japan, including me. Others were Dr. Takeshi Hirayama, Dr. Takaharu Hayashi and Dr. Sato. No one from our government. For four days from June 18 to 21 many problems concerning tobacco were presented and discussed at length. We were honored to be welcomed by the Mayor of Stockholm at a big City Hall where Nobel prizes are presented every year to outstanding men of science and literature. I was also impressed by the bulky Surgeon General's report on Smoking and Health presented to every participant as a gift from the American Surgeon General, Dr. Joseph A. Califano, who gave us a special speech. I learned for the first time that President John Kennedy in 1963 ordered the investigation of and annual reports on smoking to protect the health of the American people, with more than ten volumes of reports published by 1979. As a result, more than thirty million smokers quit smoking in the past ten years. What a contrast to Japan!

Sir George Young, the Minister of Health in Prime Minister Margaret Thatcher's administration, spoke as a representative of Great Britain. He told us how Dr. Richard Doll of Oxford University investigated the relationship of smoking to lung cancer after World War II. The accumulated evidence of the hazards of smoking persuaded physicians and volunteer groups to fight against smoking and the powerful tobacco industry. I learned later from *The Smoke Ring* written by Peter Taylor that Sir George was transferred from his post in the Department of Health to another position, shortly after this world conference, because his speech incited the rage of the tobacco industry.

# 30

# THE PRESIDENTIAL CUP

I had been the consultant to the table tennis club for medical students for many years until I resigned from my medical school. I was not, however, a table tennis player in my school days. I was a slow runner in the athletic meetings of my primary school. In the middle school in Nagasaki, I belonged to a volleyball club but was not a good player. In Saga High School there was no volleyball club and I became a member of the club of *kendo*, Japanese fencing, but I was never active, especially after three surgical operations for appendicitis and its complications. Therefore, I had never intended to practise table tennis seriously.

Yes, I played table tennis, or ping-pong, occasionally in my internship in the Ureshino Hospital, but I enjoyed playing volleyball once a week with other doctors and nurses more. After I joined the Second Department of Surgery in the University Hospital, I had the chance to play table tennis with other young residents in an abandoned surgery room. However, it was in the residents' quarter in Portland, Oregon, that I played ping-pong nearly every night with other residents after the end of our duty. I was a poor player at first, but by the end of the second year I improved my skill in table tennis and did not lose the game so easily.

Since I came back to Nagasaki from Oregon, I was too busy in neurosurgery and played table tennis only occasionally with students. I could win sometimes when I played with new club members, but it did not take long for them to beat me, for they practised daily. It was after I moved to Rosai Hospital in Sasebo that I often played table tennis during the lunch hour with young technicians and nurses. The gymnasium in the rehabilitation unit was free for the use of employees during lunch hour. A number of us had to play on the two ping-pong tables. There was no time to practise. We played games in turn. Yet the daily short play improved my skill in table tennis. I was then in my middle fifties.

It was fortunate that my next workplace, Yahata Hospital, also had one ping-pong table in an unused, small room. There were a few good table tennis players among the technicians and pharmacists of the Yahata Hospital. They were good trainers for me. After we moved to the new hospital building, we enjoyed table tennis during the short lunch hour in a conference room.

Six city hospitals in Kita-kyushu played volley ball and table tennis tournaments every spring. Each team had to include a player older than fifty years, and I had the chance to play as a member of the Yahata Hospital team every year. The Yahata Hospital team often became the winner among the six hospital teams in the city. As the best of the hospital teams we had to compete with twenty-three other departments of the city in the annual sports meeting in autumn.

We were beaten for the first few years, but we won in 1980 after beating the other twenty-three teams. I was tossed in the air by our excited team members. In the next year we won again. My partner of the doubles game was Mr. Yamasaki, a clerk from our hospital. He was not only a good player but also a good guy, who always encouraged me with his confident smile even when I missed in the game. We lost no games and were known as invincible doubles players until he left our Hospital and moved to another department of the city. However, in the singles tournament I have never been a winner, because there were many better players among the senior players over 35 and veterans over 45 years.

Good news came. The Japan Medical Association announced that it was adding table tennis to the sports events at the National Assembly of Japanese Physicians, which was held once every four years. Tennis, golf, rugby, soccer, *kendo*, and archery were other activities on the program. At the next meeting, the 21st, to be held at Osaka in 1983, the table tennis tournament was to be played in five age groups. The oldest age group was over 65, and I would reach the age of 65 on the fourth of January in 1983! I would be the youngest in the Old Veterans group. It meant that I would have a good chance to win in the oldest age group. I mailed the entry card immediately.

I was disappointed when I found the name of Professor Dennosuke Jinnai in the Old Veterans' list. Professor Jinnai was a surgeon, a graduate of Kyushu University and a former professor at Okayama University and Osaka University. He had been one of the best table tennis players in western Japan since his high school days. He was the Dean of Kinki University School of Medicine in 1983. I had read in a medical journal that he had won many medals in the past; he still played table tennis early every morning with students. The possiblity of my beating him was nil. My hope of winning was gone. There was no doubt who would be the winner. It would be Professor Jinnai, the new president of the Table Tennis Association of Medical Doctors in Japan. I suspected that he worked to have table tennis added as a new sports event at Osaka and to add the oldest age group of Old Veterans, because he was already over 65 years. He would win as he planned. What should I do? Yes, I will go and play, I told myself, for to play together is more important than to win the game. And I practised hard in the meantime.

In the evening of April 9, the new Association of Table Tennis Playing Doctors was formed, and many doctors came to the dinner party at Hotel Totenko near the Temma Bridge, Osaka. I met Professor Jinnai, who looked well, although his hair was gray. We talked about our common friends and about surgery for epilepsy, his favorite topic. My fighting spirit was gone. I had no desire to play games against Dr. Jinnai.

The day of the tournament was April 10. The games were played at a sports center called Kamiroku, a modest table tennis hall. Probably a better gymnasium was not available on such a good Sunday in the cherry blossom season.

One hundred and thirty-five doctors fought in the table tennis games, and many of them were from Osaka Prefecture: 51 from Osaka City, including 26 from Osaka University School of Medicine and 14 members of Osaka Table Tennis Club. I was the only participant from Fukuoka Prefecture.

Twenty-four teams in total played in the tournaments. Single games were played in each age group: 76 players in the age group under 35, 30 Semi-seniors of age 35 to 44, 20 Seniors of age 45 to 54, 6 Veterans over age 55, and 6 Old Veterans over age 65.

My first opponent was Professor Wada, who had defeated Dr. Kikuchi. He was 65 years old, as I was. It was an easy game for me. Professor Wada could not return my curved service ball. He gained only five points in the first game and eleven in the second match.

Fortunately I did not have to play against Professor Jinnai, because he lost the game to Dr. Higashi, age 67. Professor Jinnai, at 70 years of age, was not strong enough and could not run fast in his play. Dr. Ching defeated Dr. Higashi. The final match was Dr. Ching versus me.

Dr. Ching had been the winner in the big table tennis contest among physicians, dentists and pharmacists in Osaka. He attacked me with his unique service and speedy smash ball. He was winning at first, but my curved ball gained points in the latter half of the game. The score was 21 to 15. In the second game he returned my service ball with skill, but he missed his smashes so often that I won at last. The score was 21 to 12.

I fought desperately during the games. When all was finished, I could hardly believe that I was the winner. I would have lost the game if I had had to play against Professor Jinnai, because of my "inferiority complex." I was fortunate that I had played with a stranger. Dr. Ching was obviously confused by that strange curved ball of mine. His confidence was shaken by his own unexpected failures. Anyway, it was an unexpected victory for me.

I could not believe my victory. I wondered if I was in a dream when Professor Jinnai presented me with the commendation and the Golden Cup in the name of the President of the 21st National Assembly of Japanese Doctors. It took time to convince me of the fact that I had won.

On the way back to Kita-kyushu, I happened to meet Dr. Sakurai and other representative members of the Kita-kyushu Medical Association on the platform of Osaka Station. They hailed my victory as if they won the game. I was later asked to write about the event in the *Kita-kyushu Medical Journal.*

I confess, however, that this was my first and last victory in the table tennis tournament as a singles player. The All Japan Table Tennis Tournament for Doctors became an annual event after the first one in Osaka, but the next year I was defeated by Dr. Tai, a Formosan physician practising in Tokyo, who had been a skilled player since his days in medical school. He is the vice-president of the Table Tennis Society of Formosans in the Kanto Area. He is an expert in table tennis and I had, and will have, no chance to win against him.

The Vice President of the Doctors' Table Tennis Association was Dr. Jiro Kikuchi of Kaisei Hospital in Osaka. He was a kind gentleman and urged me to visit his hospital where he used to play with his employees. I visited him once or twice and played table tennis with him and his employees. Some of them had been champions in their school days. I enjoyed their warm hospitality as well as the ping-pong games we played.

Another earnest ping-pong loving doctor in Osaka is Dr. H. Kuriyama, who is the chief of the Doctors' Table Tennis Club in Osaka. He has his own otolaryngology clinic in Kadoma City and a private small gymnasium for table tennis behind his house, where he teaches table tennis to his friends and neighbors. I was once invited to the gymnasium and played table tennis with other medical doctors who used to play after their clinical work was finished for the day. I won games with these doctors, but not with Dr. Kuriyama, who uses a special rubber on his bat.

Every year he attends the World Athletic Meeting of Doctors, somewhere in Europe. He has won the table tennis championship twice already. He persuaded me to attend the meeting with him in 1986. I went to Monte Catini Therme, Italy, with him and his wife. Miwa came with me. I played in the singles matches in the over 40 age group. Dr. Kuriyama won the gold medal and I won the silver. We fully enjoyed our visit to Florence and Pisa during our one week tour of Italy on our way to and from Monte Catini Therme.

# 31

# WINNIPEG MANITOBA: A LETTER FROM THE CONFERENCE

"I am now in Winnipeg, Canada. I came to Winnipeg to attend an international meeting which started on July 10, 1983. It is the 5th World Conference on Smoking and Health, a big convention attended by more than one thousand individuals from eighty countries who want to make our world free from harmful tobacco smoke.

Winnipeg is not a familiar name for us Japanese. It is located in Manitoba, the central province of Canada. They claim the city is in the center of the North American Continent. The population of the city is over 600,000. Many of them are engaged in agriculture, producing wheat and corn. It looks like a big town in farming country rather than a city. The roads are wide and straight. The houses are not crowded in the city and there are only a few tall buildings in sight.

The hot climate surprised me after my flight from the cool city of Vancouver. The average highest summer temperature in daytime is 28°C and it reaches 30°C sometimes. It is too warm outdoors, while indoors the air conditioning makes it too cool. I sneezed and coughed often.

I could not understand at first why Winnipeg was selected as the place of this conference, but I can see now that the new Convention Center of the city is big enough for this mammoth conference. It has a large hall with room for more than one thousand seats. There are also a number of conference rooms of different size in addition to a cafeteria. The Center is connected to the fifteen-story Holiday Inn on the other side of the street through a corridor bridge on the second floor. I checked into this Holiday Inn, after being disappointed at the distance of another hotel which had been reserved for me. I disliked walking a long way under the scorching sun in this big town to and from the Convention Center. I was quite satisfied with the Holiday Inn. It was not only close to the Convention Center but also clean with many non-smoking floors.

In Kita-kyushu City a new building is under construction. It is the Kosei Nenkin Hall to be opened before long in the center of the city, not far from the City Office. The biggest hall will have two thousand seats. And there will be five smaller conference rooms, and enough hotel rooms for 150 guests. It is an ideal convention center, and this is one of the reasons why I considered having the next World Conference on Smoking and Health in Kita-kyushu.

Past conferences were held in New York, London, and Stockholm. All in Europe or North America, including Winnipeg. A conference should be held also in Asia, particularly in Japan where this big issue of smoking has never been discussed seriously by the nation. It is no wonder that Dr. Hirayama suggested that the next meeting be held in Japan.

If Japan is selected as the country to have the next Conference, Tokyo should be the city of choice, because it is the capital of Japan and the center of politics and business in the nation. Therefore, I was surprised when Dr. Hirayama phoned me in the middle of June asking me to come to Tokyo to meet with members of three major health organizations. He found that it was difficult to have the Conference in Tokyo. Kita-kyushu was the city of his second choice.

I went to Tokyo and asked for the support of major health groups to have the Conference in Kita-kyushu. Dr. Hirayama sent a telegram and a letter to Dr. Reed of UICC, International Union Against Cancer, telling him of our intention to invite the Conference to Japan. It was only two weeks before we left for Winnipeg. I told our intention to the board members of the Kyushu Anti-Smoking Society as soon as I came back to Kita-kyushu and all of them promised their cooperation. I also met Dr. Sonoda, the head of the Health Department of Kita-kyushu, who agreed with our plan and promised his support. I wanted to get the approval of the Mayor, but instead I asked Dr. Sonoda to inform the Mayor of the plan and ask his help, because the Mayor was too busy to see me on short notice. I told myself I could meet him after our plan is accepted by the Liaison Committee of the Conference.

In the afternoon of July 9, one day before the Conference, I was allowed to speak for fifteen minutes to the Liaison Committee in a room of the Convention Center. After Dr. Hirayama, a member of the Liaison Committee, introduced me, I explained why the next Conference should be held in Japan, where lung cancer deaths are increasing at an astonishing rate along with increasing cigarette consumption, because nothing to control smoking had been done by the government and people are not yet aware of the dangers of smoking due to a lack of information on smoking. I described our campaign in Kita-kyushu since 1977 and the wish of our members to have a successful conference in Japan. I gave information about the city of Kita-kyushu as a candidate city with its hotel capacity, transportation and other attractions to host participants from all over the world. Dr. Hirayama added a few explanations about the attitudes of other health groups in Japan to the next conference. The committee was to vote for the place of the next conference after hearing the reports of other candidate nations, and the final decision was to be announced on the last day of the Congress.

There was a colorful, exciting welcome party on the evening of July 9 at the Centennial Hall. People from different countries paraded on the main street to the Hall from the Convention Center under the scorching sun, but all discomfort was compensated for by the glamour of the party. Panoramic views of many different regions in Canada were projected onto the huge screen. Then men and women in different national costumes demonstrated their unique dances on the stage, representing various nationalities of the immigrants to Canada. I enjoyed, above all, the Cossack dances of the Ukrainian descendants. The dances were fascinating and the smiles of the beautiful girls were charming. At the end there was a standing ovation. In my mind I wondered what kind of entertainment we could offer in Kita-kyushu, if the same audience gathered there four years later.

The World Conference started on Monday, July 11. The Honorable Monique Begin, Canadian Minister of National Health and Welfare, gave us her welcome address. The message of Dr. Halfdan Mahler, Director-General of the World Health Organization, was read by a delegate from WHO. Sir George Godber, the former British Minister of Health, reviewed the history of the World

Conference over 16 years and congratulated us all for our concern and achievement in the past.

Plenary presentations were given by Dr. Jesse L. Steinfeld of U.S.A.and Dr. Nigel Gray of Australia. The former spoke on "The Harmful Health Consequences of Smoking" and the latter on "The Socio-economic Implications of Tobacco." In the afternoon, Dr. Mary Jane Ashley of Canada spoke on "Smoking and Women," and Dr. Theodor Abelin of Switzerland on "Smoking of Children." Both of them were concerned about the present trends in smoking. The only good news was the decline of smoking rates among American teenagers, proving the effects of an active campaign. The rates of smoking among the adult population dropped in the United States from 41 percent to 32 percent in males and from 32 percent to 29 percent in females over the last fifteen years. The smoking rate of Japanese women is much lower at the present time, but we must keep watching the growing number of female smokers in Japan. After their presentations I had a chance to talk with the presenters personally for one hour.

The plenary presentation on the next day, July 12, was given by Dr. Kjell Bjartveit of Norway. It was a grand speech. In Norway, since the first comprehensive national tobacco legistation in the world was set up in 1975, all kinds of tobacco promotion were forbidden, smoking in public places was restricted, and education on smoking was given to all children and students. As a result, smoking among young people decreased drastically and non-smoking generations are growing in this tobacco-conscious nation.

In the afternoon concurrent sessions started in nine rooms. I listened to the topics on legislation in Room 1. The experience of the "Minnesota Clean Indoor Air Act" reported by Jeanne Weigum was as interesting as the result of legislation in Norway. Smoking was banned in restaurants and coffee shops in Minnesota, except in limited smoking areas. Non-smoking is the norm in Minnesota and Norway. It is interesting that 70 to 80 percent of smokers welcomed the law, according to surveys following the legislation. Japan should learn from their examples. Smoking should be banned in all restaurants in Kita-kyushu, if the next Conference were to be held in that city.

There were so many sessions going at the same time that it was hard to decide which session I should attend. I had to move from one room to another to listen to the most interesting speeches. The common opinions from many sessions can be summarized as follows:

*1. All advertising and promotion of tobacco should be prohibited.*
*2. Legislation is urgently needed to ban smoking from all public places including transportion, the workplace, government offices and hospitals.*
*3. Education on smoking should be mandatory in schools and communities.*
*4. The tax and price of cigarettes should be raised and the profit should be spent on education about smoking.*
*5. Teachers and parents should be non-smoking models for children.*
*6. Medical Associations should lead the actions listed above.*
*7. The warning on cigarette packages should state that "Smoking is the main cause of cancer, heart diseases and other illness."*

Japanese participants in this World Conference were shamefully few. Only eleven in total from Japan, a nation of 120 million population! Besides Dr. Hirayama and me there were Mr. Kenji Makino, a correspondent from the Mainichi Newspaper and the author of Tobaccology, Dr. Hiroshi Ogawa from Aichi Cancer Center, Dr. Takaharu Hayashi of the Tokyo Eisei Hospital, Dr. Morizo Sakihara from Okinawa, Dr. Toshio Nibu from Iwakuni City, Dr. and Mrs. Igarashi of Toyama N.S. Club, Lawyer Isayama, Mr. Bungaku Watanabe of the Ken-En-Ken group, and Rev. Miyazaki, a Seventh Day Adventist. We met at the Oriental Restaurant one evening and discussed the future anti-smoking strategy for Japan.

My presentation was on the afternoon of July 14. The chairman of the session on community programs was Dr. Adam Tahy, my Hungarian friend. For twenty minutes I talked on "The Progress and Problems of the Anti-Smoking Movement in Japan." The presence of Japanese in the audience relaxed me. I reported on the progress of the non-smoking movement in Japan since 1977 and the result in Kita-kyushu. The tobacco industry has been a monopoly of the Japanese government, bringing a large income to the government. It is the Japanese government which neglected to enlarge non-smoking areas in trains and public places, which never interfered with tobacco advertising and promotion, which was indifferent about education on smoking and health both in schools and communities.

My report on the success of education in Yahata High School surprised the audience. After concentrated education on smoking for one year, only two new smokers were added to the twelve previous smokers among 400 students, and none of the girls smoked, while smoking rates of teenage girls in other nations are as high as 30 percent or more.

One of our problems is smoking among the medical professions. The rate is still over 30 percent, not much different from 35 percent in Hungary, whereas only about 10 percent of doctors in England, Australia and the United States smoke now.

There were many presentations on smoking among women. I can understand that uneducated women receiving social welfare smoke more than other women, but it was a surprise to hear that smoking is not uncommon among nurses, higher than 30 percent in some countries. Smoking among children seemed much higher in other countries than in Japan, but the result of intensive education on smoking in the State of Minnesota was remarkable. Japan should follow this example, but it will be difficult in Japan where 59 percent of teachers smoke.

Tomorrow is the last day of the Conference. The name of the city which hosts the next Conference will be announced tomorrow. I will report on it later." (July 14, 1983 at Winnipeg)

My report to the Kita-kyushu Medical Association ended there. This letter was printed in the September issue of *The Journal of Kita-kyushu Medical Association*, followed by a copy of a Mainichi newspaper report:

"The 6th World Conference on Smoking and Health will be held in Kita-kyushu in 1987. The decision was announced on July 15 at the end of the 5th World Conference on Smoking and Health at Winnipeg, Canada. Dr. Takeshi Hirayama, the chief epidemiologist of the National Cancer Institute, was nominated as President. The chairman of the program committee will be Dr. Martin M. Kawano, Director of the Yahata City Hospital in Kita-kyushu. The announcement of this decision was welcomed by a standing ovation. This World Conference is held every four years to discuss the problems of smoking and health from medical, social, economic, and many other standpoints among health professionals and citizens aiming at the goal of reducing the harmful influence of smoking on health around the world. At the Liaison Committee meeting in the evening of July 14, Japan was selected as the next host nation to hold the 6th Conference" (reported by Makino at Winnipeg, Canada).

# 32

# THE ANTI-SMOKING REVOLUTION

Dr. Takeshi Hirayama is well known all over the world. Many speakers in Winnipeg referred to the statistical data of his study. When he spoke in a session, the room was full and many questions and discussions followed his speech. It was no wonder, because his outstanding follow-up study of 265,118 Japanese for many years has been highly acclaimed throughout the world. The World Health Organization appointed him as a member of its committee on smoking. His epidemiological data are cited in the Report of the WHO Expert Committee "Smoking and its Effects on Health"(1975), "Controlling the Smoking Epidemic"(1979) and many other publications.

I invited Dr. Hirayama for the first time to Kita-kyushu in the spring of 1980. He spoke at two meetings, one for the general public and another for medical doctors. His straight, precise approach to the problem and his patriotic passion for the improvement of the long-neglected, serious menace of smoking in Japan impressed all the audience. I asked him to stay overnight in our apartment house in Yahata. Early next morning, I took him to the city water reservoir on a hill, because it was the cherry blossom season. Dr. Hirayama brought a sketch-book with him, and he sketched the beautiful cherry trees on its pages, paying no attention to the drops of rain falling upon him. I was surprised at his love for beauty and his readiness to preserve it on paper, while I held an umbrella to protect him from the rain.

One morning, a year later, I was surprised by big bundles of letters delivered to my office. All the letters were from people asking me to mail my booklet *Dangerous Tobacco Pollution.* They had learned about the booklet from a column called "Prism" in the *Asahi* newspaper.

"Prism" is written by Mrs. Yukiko Ohkuma, who belongs to the Science Section of the *Asahi* newspaper. On the previous Saturday, May 23, 1981, she wrote a short report under the title "The Dangers of Smoking." She wrote on the death of my niece as a victim of smoking and introduced my booklet, which I was trying to distribute. The address of the Yahata Hospital was added at the end. I remembered a telephone call I had received a few days before. The lady on the telephone asked me, in her polite Tokyo accent, about the lung cancer deaths of my relatives. She was Mrs. Ohkuma, I discovered. Her refined vocabulary and charming voice were quite different from those of the journalists I had previously known. I could hardly believe that she was a journalist.

I had to mail the booklets day after day. Miwa's help was not enough. I hired two girls to help us. The stock of booklets did not last long. I ordered more copies, but the capacity of a small printing shop is limited. I had to apologize daily, by telephone and in postcards, for the delay of our mailing. It was a month before we were able to cope with the flood of orders. Our efforts, however, were worthwhile because many people in distant parts of Japan, such as Hokkaido, the Northeast and Okinawa, read my booklet on smoking and realized the risk of tobacco and the serious pollution of the air by its smoke. The single voice of my warning will not lead to enlarged non-smoking areas in trains, airlines, and restaurants unless public awareness is raised by people who became aware of the hazards of smoking. I was impressed by the big influence of mass media demonstrated in this month. Even one small column of a newspaper can get a big response from the public. I should appeal more often through the newspapers and other mass media. I hope more and more people write letters to the newspapers emphasizing the need for control of and education on smoking, using the summarized information I presented to thousands of individuals in Japan.

After the turmoil of the "Prism" came an unexpected request from a publisher named Bunsen. I was asked to write a book under the title *The Dangers of Smoking*. The publisher must have heard of the reactions to the article by Mrs. Ohkuma. Bunsen is not a big publisher, but I thought it was a good opportunity to write down many more facts about smoking which I could not include in my small booklet. I agreed to meet an editor of the publisher when I went to Tokyo to attend the international conference on cerebral hemorrhage. Mr. Niikawa was a polite gentleman, and I found him reliable and capable. As I expected, he edited a handsome book with a fine red cover of good design. The first edition was published on March 3, 1982. Dr. Hirayama wrote an introduction for the book under the title, "Read through and act upon it!" from which I include the following excerpt:

*Tragedies are happening around you. Smokers are dying one after another due to tobacco diseases. Prime Minister Ikeda and Prime Minister Ohira would still have been alive and active if they had never smoked. Passive smoking can also increase the risk of lung cancer death. It is true that most Japanese are now suffering from varying degrees of tobacco diseases.*

*In order to understand the facts about tobacco diseases, read this book. You will hear the sincere voice of Dr. Kawano speaking directly to your heart. You will see a man standing against the smoking epidemic and trying to combat it with his hands and body and soul.*

Assisted by Dr. Hirayama's encouraging introduction, this new book written by an unknown author sold well and was reprinted. One evening, many friends of mine in Kita-kyushu gathered at the Kokura Station Hotel to celebrate the publication of my new book. Dr. Sakurai, president of the Kita-kyushu Medical Association, was one of the guests. Professor Wakizaka came from Kurume and gave a congratulatory speech. So many members of the Medical Association and of the Kyushu Antismoking Society came to this dinner party and congratulated me that I did not know how to thank them all. I thanked God for my good fortune in finding so many kind acquaintances in Kita-kyushu, where I hardly knew anyone five years ago. Mr. Tani, Mayor of the City, appeared in the middle of the party and gave a kind greeting to us all. His wife was also present. I dreamed of the day when he would make public his idea of creating a "Smoke-free City" in Kita-kyushu.

A new wing was added to the Yahata Hospital before I left for Winnipeg. The new construction started in August, 1981 because the previous 240 beds were not enough for the ever-increasing number of patients, many of whom were emergency cases. The space for the new wing was reserved from the beginning of the first construction to be available for future expansion. This time there was no such inconvenience for the patients as we had had in the earlier building process. Not only were additional wards for patients built but also a new rehabilitation center in the new wing. More rooms were added for x-ray examination, clinical pathology, conference, a medical library, and doctors' quarters. The new building cost as much as the first building, but the city was willing to pay the cost because the need was urgent. When the new 400-bed hospital was completed, the Mayor came to see the new building and to offer congratulations at the celebration party. The new wing was opened in September. The new intensive care unit had 14 beds. The fourth floor of the new wing with fifty beds and much modern equipment was used exclusively for emergency cases. No longer did we wake up other patients on other floors as we brought in the emergency cases at night, because all new emergency cases could be hospitalized on this floor until moved to other floors in the daytime, depending on their diagnosis. I thanked the Mayor for the new construction and expected him to support us in the coming 6th World Conference on Smoking and Health in 1987.

At the New Year's speech in 1984, Mayor Tani called the attention of the city employees to the World Conference to be held in 1987. Later, he called me to his office with a question and some advice: "How is it going with your preparation for the World Conference? You should not waste time, because time flies fast. You must be well prepared. You should consult with the head of our Health Department."

In fact, the preparation was blocked by obstacles. After coming back from Canada, I had no call from Dr. Hirayama until December. I thought he was too busy running around the world, but I wondered if anything was wrong. It was in December when I was asked to come to Tokyo to meet the representatives of three major health organizations and the Ministry of Health and Welfare. The air of the meeting was tense. Breaking the silence, Dr. Shimao of the Japan Anti-Tuberculosis Association blamed Dr. Hirayama and me bluntly:

"Why, and in what kind of capacity, did you invite the next World Conference to Japan? We have not yet agreed to have the next Conference in Japan, although the Heart Foundation is for it. We have never appointed you to represent the leading health groups in Japan. We also want to know why you have neglected to inform us on the final decision after coming back from the last Conference in Canada."

He requested us further to report in letters to the concerned health bodies in Japan, the Japanese government and to the Mayor of Kita-kyushu all the steps leading to Japan's selection as the next host of the Conference. That was the end of the meeting.

They met again in 1984, on February 1 and on May 17, at the office of the Anti-Tuberculosis Association in Tokyo, but Dr. Hirayama and I were not invited. All I learned from the letter of Mr. Yoshioka, Secretary General of the Japan Heart Foundation, was that the Mayor of Kita-kyushu had spoken with Mr. Kitani, the assistant director of the Foundation, who visited the Mayor's office in March. "If the three major health organizations and the Ministry of Health and Welfare reach agreement and ask the City of Kita-kyushu to join, we are ready to join you. We shall open an office in the City Hall and co-operate with our branch in Tokyo."

Therefore, it was a surprise to hear the announcement of Dr. Motomura,the newly appointed director of the City Department of Health, in April, "The World Conference on Smoking and Health should be sponsored by civic groups. The City will not give any help. We have no intention of becoming a sponsor."

A few days later Mrs. Tomiyasu and I were asked to come to the Health Department in the City Hall. We were told, "We have not yet had a written request from you to assist the World Conference on Smoking and Health. There is no official record of it and we have no intention of spending any money on the Conference." I was appalled but said nothing.

I was not the only one who was surprised at the sudden change in the City's attitude. Dr. Tadao Shimao wrote in his letter to the Mayor dated October 18:

*The three health bodies in Japan had believed that your city would actively sponsor the World Conference as soon as we reached agreement among our groups. However, when we invited one of the officials from your Health Department, the Executive Manager of the Department told us that the issue of the World Conference had never been discussed in the Department, which knew nothing about the Conference and is not yet at the stage to discuss sponsorship. This statement shocked all of us who represented the three bodies.*

On July 19, Dr. Motomura went to Tokyo and explained to each group: (1) It is difficult for the City to be a sponsor of the Conference. (2) We can consider opening the local headquarters in the City Hall. (3) The capacity of the hotels in Kita-kyushu is not large enough to accommodate the Conference.

Dr. Shimao visited Kita-kyushu on August 23 but could not meet the Mayor. He wrote to the Mayor again on September 7, asking if the city was willing to become a sponsor. The answer came by telephone from the Health Department. The City refused again for the reason that hotel rooms and good Western-style restaurants were insufficient to accommodate so many guests from overseas.

Dr. Tominaga of Aichi Cancer Institute told me in a letter that it might be necessary to change the place of the Conference to Tokyo if it were difficult to have it in Kita-kyushu because of the city's lack of cooperation.

In a letter of October 18, Dr. Shimao asked me to come to Tokyo and discuss the final decision. He presented the following options for consideration:

Plan 1. The Kyushu Anti-Smoking Society sponsors the Conference in Kita-kyushu with the help of the City.

Plan 2. Dr. Hirayama and Dr. Kawano inform the Liaison Committee that they cannot organize the Conference in Japan.

Plan 3. Three major health bodies organize the Conference in Tokyo, if the above two plans are difficult.

I went to Tokyo on November 16 as I was ordered. The meeting started at 2:00 p.m. in the conference room of the Anti-Tuberculosis Association. Members representing three health groups and the Ministry of Health and Welfare were there. Dr. Motomura and his assistant represented the Health Department of Kita-kyushu City. Dr. Hirayama could not come on time, but I knew his principles, which were:

1. The Conference will be held in Kita-kyushu as we decided.

2. It is up to the three major health groups whether or not they sponsor the Conference.

3. The main sponsor should be the civic anti-smoking group.

4. The Conference will be limited to the problems of smoking, in spite of possible pressure from any authority, either the government or the tobacco industry.

The meeting started in a tense mood. Mr. Yoshioka of the Heart Foundation was the Chairman. Following his report on the past negotiations, Dr. Motomura apologized for the reluctance of Kita-kyushu City to sponsor the Conference. I explained the situation in Winnipeg, where Dr. Hirayama was named as the President to organize the next World Conference, and added Dr. Hirayama's ideas, which I supported. Sharp questions followed my report, as I expected.

"Dr. Hirayama and the Kyushu Anti-smoking Society invited the next World Conference to Japan without the full agreement of the three major health groups. Are you ready to carry the responsibility of your invitation?"

"Yes, I will. Even if the City of Kita-kyushu refuses to help us, we shall open the World Conference in Kita-kyushu. We ask you to help us as much as you can."

Dr. Motomura stood up again and interfered, "I say again, gentlemen. 0ur city has no intention to sponsor or to give any help to the World Conference!"

"We shall carry on our plan without any help from the City," I had to tell him. Silence governed the room after my words. At last Mr. Yoshioka broke the silence.

"The Japan Heart Foundation will do our best to help you."

The meeting was over. On the way to Haneda Airport, I stopped at the Asahi Newspaper Building and met Mrs.Yukiko Ohkuma, who had been promoted to membership on the editorial board. "It seems that things did not happen as Dr. Shimao expected. Maybe it was good after all." She consoled me.

The Japanese Ministry of Health and Welfare did not think that it was good. Dr. Gunji of the Section of Health Promotion and Nutrition was deeply concerned about our difficult situation. He asked Dr. Hirayama and me to discuss the problem with him, On February 6 of the next year, I went to the National Cancer Institute to join Dr. Hirayama and Dr. Tominaga. We went together to the Ministry of Health and Welfare.

Dr. Gunji is a graduate of the Tokyo University School of Medicine. He played in the orchestra in which Mrs. Ohkuma played the piano as a student. He was a polite gentleman with good manners. He invited us to lunch at a nearby restaurant. He asked us to give him a free hand to organize a new body to sponsor the World Conference by coordinating the efforts of the Ministry of Health and Welfare, the three major health groups and the Health Promotion Foundation. He explained the need for a new scientific organization on smoking and health. Such an organization could get support and subsidies from the government, which would be freed from ownership of the Tobacco Monopoly Corporation by the next April. However, the total stocks of the new company, Japan Tobacco Co. (JT), have been held by the Minister of Finance until now.

I heard nothing from Tokyo after the agreement was made between Dr. Hirayama and Dr. Gunji. More than six months after our meeting, an *Asahi Newspaper* reporter in Kita-kyushu interviewed me at the Yahata Hospital. I learned from him that the World Conference would be held in the Keidanren Building, Tokyo, from November 9 to 11, in 1987. I frankly told him of my regret that Kita-kyushu was no longer the candidate city to hold the Conference because the City refused to sponsor the Conference.

The situation had changed suddenly when the new Chief of the City Department of Health, Dr. Motomura, replaced Dr. Sonoda, who had encouraged me to invite the Conference to Kita-kyushu. A lack of hotel capacity is not a convincing reason to turn down the World Conference which the Mayor was once in favor of. The main reason must be a financial one, because I heard that Dr. Sonoda was flatly refused by the Financial Department of the City when he asked for a budget to prepare for the Conference.

My suspicion was confirmed when I found out the figures for the tobacco tax revenue of the city; 4,764,580,000 yen in 1984, or more than 35,000,000 dollars in one year (if $1=135yen)! The city knows that my booklet *Dangerous Tobacco Pollution* reduced the consumption of cigarettes in the city by more than five percent in 1977-1978. The city cannot afford to sponsor an international congress on smoking and health, which will surely reduce the sales of tobacco products and consequently the huge sales tax.

The Department of Commerce was willing to help us, because hundreds of visitors to the Conference from abroad would bring in good customers to the city and fill vacancies in hotel rooms and restaurants. It would be devastating, however, for the Financial Department of the City, which would have to face the reduction in tobacco sales tax, not only temporarily but constantly if the Conference were to convince the citizens of the dangers of smoking. Even if the Mayor were enthusiastic, the city officials would be against the scheme for obvious financial reasons. Now I understood all. Nevertheless, I should be content that the Conference would be held in Japan after all, in Tokyo, the capital of Japan, even if not in Kita-kyushu. As the one who worked to invite the Conference to Japan I should be satisfied. It was good for our nation that we had worked for the nomination of Japan as the host of the next World Conference on Smoking and Health.

Next morning, the *Asahi* newspaper reported the interview with a big headline in the local news: "Anti-Smoking Olympics has gone with a puff of smoke—No more in Kita-kyushu," "Is Tobacco Tax more valuable than Health? Anti-Smoking Congress in Kita-kyushu given up."

The article which followed cited my answers to the interviewer, which explained that the cancellation was due to the change of attitude of city officials concerned with revenue. The director of the tax office told the reporter, "A tobacco tax of 4,764,000,000 yen is certainly a stable, easily-earned tax income for the city, and we have campaigned in the past to encourage citizens to buy more tobacco in our city. However, we did not oppose either the non-smokers-rights movement or the anti-smoking convention."

As I anticipated, the city reacted to this news immediately. The Department of Hospital Administration demanded me to come to the office. As soon as I arrived at the office, the Director ordered me to apologize to the Mayor for my statement in the newspaper. As I walked side by side with the Director of the Department toward the Mayor's office, I decided to resign my job as the Superintendent of the Yahata Hospital. I knew I was no longer needed in this city.

I presented my resignation to the Mayor on the first of December, and retired on December 28, the last working day of 1986. No one tried to stop me.

The French revolution started in 1789. If you reverse the last three numbers, the year 1987 would be the year when the anti-smoking revolution was ignited in Japan. Norway started in 1975 to launch a national campaign to bring up "Non-Smoking Generations." The American Medical Association has announced its target of "Smoke-free 2000." I was impressed in Scotland by the campaign called "Glasgow 2000," when I was invited to speak during the "Health Week" of the city in the summer of 1984.

As the common people fought against the ruler and ended the rule of the Nobles in the French revolution, it is high time for non-smokers to reform the nation and society of Japan by resisting the rulers of the tobacco industry.

Smoking should be prohibited in Japanese workplaces as it is in San Francisco and many other cities in the United States. Smoking should be banned from all public places and transportation, as in New York. Smoking should be prohibited in all official buildings, as in the United States. It is only logical to forbid smoking in hospitals, schools, trains, airplanes, restaurants, and many other places in the presence of non-smokers. If these common sense and healthy rules guide our society, all diseases related to smoking will decrease and disappear at last, not only cancers of all organs, coronary heart diseases, and chronic bronchial diseases, but also many other diseases, anomalies, miscarriages and mental deficiencies. Everyone can enjoy smokefree, clean, unpolluted air in their communities. I prayed that 1987 would be the year for Japan to inaugurate an anti-smoking revolution toward a smoke-free new world.

In the spring of 1987, the names of the organizing committee members of the World Conference were announced. The President was Mr. Yoshizane Iwasa of the Japan Heart Foundation. Secretary General was Dr. Suketami Tominaga. Other members consisted of representative members of three major health groups in Japan. The Conference would be a successful one, because the Japan Medical Association and big businessmen were committed to support it. Kita-kyushu lost the honor of being the host of the 6th World Conference on Smoking and Health, despite my hope of starting the anti-smoking revolution at Kita-kyushu in the revolutionary year of 1987. Nevertheless, I intended to organize an international symposium in Kita-kyushu for a smoke-free new century, because the anti-smoking movement in Kyushu started at Kita-kyushu with us.

# 33

# FINALE

On the 9th of November, 1987, ten years after the death of my brother, the 6th World Conference on Smoking and Health started in Tokyo. In total, 702 delegates, including 268 Japanese, gathered from 58 nations. At the opening ceremony in the Keidanren Building, I was given a seat on the stage next to Dr. Tominaga, Secretary General of the Conference. In the opening message President Iwasa introduced me as the one who worked to bring this Conference to Japan.

After the greetings by the Minister of Health and Welfare and the Mayor of Tokyo, Dr. Halfdan Mahler, Director-General of the World Health Organization, gave an address emphasizing the urgent need to fight against the serious menace of smoking in the world. Every year, more than two million people are dying as the result of smoking, and the number of victims will increase year after year owing to the rapid increase of smokers in the developing countries. He reminded the tobacco exporting nations of their responsibility.

The first Plenary lecture on the first day of the Conference was "Health Effects of Smoking" given by Dr. Hirayama. He fascinated the audience by countless graphs and figures of his epidemiological survey of 265,118 Japanese followed up for 17 years. It was a big demonstration of the recorded proof that, not only cancers of the lung and trachea, but many other malignancies, and diseases of the heart, digestive organs and respiratory organs, increase as the number of cigarettes smoked per day increases. The audience was impressed further by his data on passive smoking. The non-smoking wives of those husbands who smoked less than 19 cigarettes per day died of lung cancer 1.45 times more than non-smokers' wives, and the rate increased to 1.91 times if the husbands smoked more than twenty cigarettes per day. He introduced fifteen similar studies by other scholars in the world. One of them reported the amazing rate of 3.5 times among wives of smokers who smoked more than one pack a day. All the figures are undeniable facts, even if the tobacco industry argues that they are nothing but figures on paper. Already known are the facts that the smoking of husbands increases the risk of cancers of the nose, breast, and brain, not to mention the risk of coronary heart disease, of their wives.

Dr. Hirayama surprised the audience by his new study on the aging effect of smoking. Alzheimer's disease is common among smokers. Smoking will speed up the aging process, five years faster on the average. The incidence of all cancers and heart diseases among smokers is similar to that of non-smokers five years older. If one starts smoking earlier than age fifteen, the aging process will be 15 years faster than for non-smokers. That is why such people die of cancer an average of 15 years earlier than non-smokers. We know so many movie stars who died young, either of cancer or a heart attack. The liver is most vulnerable to tobacco. The incidence of liver cirrhosis and liver cancer is high among smokers. Smoking is far more harmful for the liver than alcohol.

By November 12, the last day of the Conference, 220 persons had presented their lectures and reports. I was the Chairman of a free talking session in the afternoon of the 10th. I also spoke during the session. I pointed out the reasons behind the extremely high rate of smoking, 62.5 per cent, among Japanese adult males. The Japanese government is responsible for the lack of education on smoking and health and for the flood of tobacco advertisements in all kinds of mass media including television. The secret reason for this might be the huge sales tax, contributing three percent of the government's income. Politicians, officials of the Ministry of Health and Welfare, physicians and school teachers share the responsibility by their indifference and bad examples of smoking. I stressed the need for legislation to control smoking in hospitals, schools, workplaces, and all public places including trains, airplanes, and other public transportation. All advertisements and promotion of tobacco should be banned immediately.

The International Symposium for a Smoke-free New Century started in Kita-kyushu on Friday, November 13. The Kita-kyushu Committee on Smoking and Health was anxious to have an international meeting in the city, even after they lost the chance of hosting the World Conference. The selection of guest speakers was my responsibility. After inviting several well-known foreign speakers devoted to a smoke-free society, I received acceptances from six Americans, one Australian, one New Zealander, and one from Scotland. Except Mr. John Gaiser of New Zealand and Miss Ruth Kendal of Glasgow, I had not met them, but all expressed their willingness to participate in our symposium. Dr. Hirayama was the only Japanese among the symposiasts. I recommended him as the President of the symposium, but I had to take this responsibility myself in consideration of the situation. Mrs. Tomiyasu worked hard to raise funds for the symposium and all the committee members cooperated with her. I am grateful to everyone who donated money to the Kyushu Anti-Smoking Society.

More than four hundred citizens came to the symposium at the Kyushu Kosei Nenkin Hall. The first speaker was Dr. Michael Daube of the Western Australia Health Department, who would be in charge of the World Conference in 1990 in Perth. He spoke on the reason why we should bring in a smoke-free new century for our children and taught us how to reach this goal. He emphasized the need for guidance from the state and cooperation of the mass media in education on smoking and health. His tones of clear, scholarly British English reminded us of his career as former professor at Edinburgh University.

Miss Ruth Kendal is an amiable woman who is actively working on the "Glasgow 2000" project. She reported on the project plan and its progress in the last four years. It will not be easy for Glasgow to save the citizens from the reign of lung cancer and coronary heart disease, because 42 percent of the women smoke as much as the men in Glasgow. Her story was interesting for me because I had visited Glasgow in 1984 as a guest of the city and received a tartan check tie from the Lord Provost.

The Great New Zealand Smoke-Free Week in June, 1986 was reported by Mr. John Gaiser from the Auckland Division of the Cancer Society of New Zealand. He amazed us with the surprising results of the event: 13 per-cent of the smokers in New Zealand stopped smoking during the week and the consumption of cigarettes dropped by 25 percent after the introduction of a higher tobacco tax which followed the week.

Dr. Leland L. Fairbanks disclosed his strategy, which succeeded in making more than two hundred hospitals belonging to the Indian Health Service smoke-free within one year. It was quite a contrast to Japanese hospitals where cigarettes are sold and smoking is permitted.

Regina Carlson had a stately figure and a good smile. She, with other citizens of the state, created a New Jersey Group Against Smoking Pollution in 1974, and has worked for years to protect non-smokers. She told us about the activities and tactics of GASP, comparing them to the action of the naive boy in the parable of the emperor's clothes.

The story of Donna Shimp was also impressive. She used to be a heavy smoker until she met her present husband, a non-smoker. After she quit smoking, she was annoyed by the smoke of her colleagues. Her protest led to a suit against the Bell Telephone Company and she won the case with the help of GASP and many other conscientious individuals. Her last words echoed in the ears of all of us in the audience: "Never...Never...Never give up!"

On the second day of the symposium Jeanne Weigum reported the circumstances under which the Minnesota Clean Indoor Air Act, the first statewide indoor air regulation, was passed in 1975. This unexpected passage of the bill was ignored at first, but is recognized now as the centerpiece of a comprehensive statewide smoking control program. She analyzed the secret of the success of the legislation for us.

The Honorable Wendy Nelder, a member of the San Francisco Board of Supervisors, wrote for the city of San Francisco the toughest American smoking ordinance ever considered before 1982. She revealed to us the interesting story of how she conceived the idea and how she fought against big opposition before the bill's dramatic passage. This first comprehensive regulation of smoking in the workplace became the model of other legislation in the United States.

Dr. Raymond D. Weisberg of ANSR (Americans for Nonsmokers' Rights) gave a comment on the passage of this ordinance from the viewpoint of a concerned citizens' group, and he told us what is happening at the federal level in the United States. He also discussed the dispute in New York on the new, severe regulations on smoking proposed by Mayor Koch.

The last speaker of the symposium was Dr. Hirayama, who demonstrated again his massive epidemiological proof of the damage resulting from passive smoking. He was as convincing as he was in the Conference in Tokyo.

At the end of the symposium, Mrs. Tomiyasu stood up and asked the audience for approval of the concluding appeals of the symposium:

1. Leaders of all kinds should set a good example to young people by not smoking.
2. Education on smoking should be started at an early age and continued to protect children from the habit of smoking.
3. All advertising and promotion of cigarettes should be prohibited by law.
4. All vending machines for cigarettes should be banned.
5. Smoking should be eliminated in schools, hospitals, government buildings and all other public places.
6. Non-smoking policies should be established in the workplace.
7. Smoking should be banned from all forms of transportation.
8. Non-smokers, children in particular, must be protected from cigarette smoke.
9. Clear, definite warnings should be printed on the packages of tobacco.
10. Taxes on tobacco products should be raised periodically.

This International Symposium in Kita-kyushu ended in success. As soon as it ended at noon, I invited the symposiasts to a bus tour of Kyushu Island. Mr. Owaku of the Heart Foundation and Mr. Bungaku Watanabe of TOPIC (Tobacco Problem Information Center) joined us. I planned to have another symposium in Oita after travelling across Kyushu Island through Nagasaki and Unzen National Park. We missed Dr. Daube and Dr. and Mrs. Weisberg, who could not travel with us.

Our first stop on the way to Nagasaki was Arita, an old town of ceramic arts. We enjoyed the exhibition of fine china wares of all kinds at the Museum of Ceramic Arts. After arriving at Nagasaki in the evening, we had a wonderful Japanese dinner party in a Japanese tatami room on the fourth floor of the Nagasaki Kosei Nenkin Hotel. The evening view of Mount Inasa was beautiful with the scarlet sky in the background. It was the first Japanese style dinner the foreign guests had enjoyed since they came to Japan. Some of them took photographs of the decorated meals on the table. There were also present some members of the Kyushu Anti-Smoking Society in Nagasaki in addition to Miwa and her niece. The wife of Professor Tsuji sat between Jeanne Weigum and me and we talked about Minneapolis and St. Paul. In their speeches Dr. Fairbanks and Donna Shimp praised my efforts in inviting the World Conference to Japan. I was glad that everyone enjoyed the evening.

Next day was Sunday. In the afternoon we visited the Glover House, a historical house from where one has the best view of the harbor, as Madame Butterfly did in a scene of Puccini's opera.

However, everyone was eager to visit the Atomic Bomb Memorial Museum built near the hypocenter in Urakami. They watched the exhibited relics and photographs of the bombing of Nagasaki with keen interest. I noticed tears in some eyes when I answered questions about my own experience at the time of the explosion.

On the way from Nagasaki to Unzen we said farewell to Donna Shimp and her husband at Nagasaki Airport. Arriving at Unzen shortly before sunset, we had the good fortune to see the sun sinking down behind the peaks of the National Park from the viewpoint of Nita Pass. It was already dark when we arrived at the Unzen International Hotel.

Our tempura dinner in a separate Japanese building of the hotel was fun. We ate each tempura as soon as it was picked up by the chef from the boiling pan in front of us. My international comrades, brave heroes and heroines who fought in the campaigns against smoking, were enjoying tempura and sake together, chatting and joking to each other while relaxing in our informal yukata kimonos. I felt as if a heavy burden was removed from my shoulders after I had borne it for a long time.

We left Unzen early the next morning. The autumn sky was all blue without a spot of cloud. Our bus drove down the slope of Mt. Unzen to the harbor of Shimabara. The big car ferry took us across Ariake Bay to Misumi Harbor. After another hour's bus ride we stood on the rim of Mt. Aso's crater. We looked down through the fume and steam of the volcano into the deep bottom of the crater. No one wanted to leave the place until I urged them to come back to our chartered bus.

We arrived at Beppu later than planned and hurried to a former Australian liner named "Oriana," where our hosts in Beppu and Oita were waiting for us with a welcome dinner party.

While I was listening to the greeting speeches of the President of the Oita Medical Association and other hosts, I thought of the final symposium scheduled on the following day in Oita City. Suddenly I felt lonesome. Tomorrow will be the end of my long journey started in 1977 with the death of my brother. I must take my leave from all the guests who came from far countries. I will miss them and all that happened in this unforgettable November in 1987. At that moment there came into my mind the closing words of General MacArthur at the end of his farewell speech to the Congress after he was dismissed from his job in Japan and South Korea,

"Old soldiers never die, they just fade away."

# PART IV

# 34

# A SNOW-WHITE MORNING

My father was a son of a fisherman in Oita Prefecture. He was born in a fishing village called Hato, which in Japanese means "dove." He went to Kobe in his youth and learned how to bake Senbei, a thin crisp rice cracker. Later, he opened a cake store selling Senbei in Nagasaki. His special brands of "Suwasenbei" and "Misosenbei" sold well, and the store became quite popular around town. By the time I entered primary school, my father had given the store to my eldest brother, who was eighteen years older than I. My father opened another small store down the same street near a stream. I lived in my father's new house on the other side of the stream, but my parents did not stay at home during the daytime; they worked in the store from early morning until late in the evening.

My parents had many children. I was the youngest of their seven sons. The second oldest brother graduated from a school of commerce but wanted to be a teacher. He finally became a primary school teacher in Sasebo, 80km from Nagasaki. The third brother loved painting and left home in his youth to become a painter. The fourth brother was a quiet man. He stayed with my father and helped him around the store. One day in summer he felt a pain in his abdomen but kept working until it was too late. His inflamed appendix burst and fatal peritonitis developed. He died shortly after emergency surgery. He was only 22 years old. He loved me and cared for me most among my six brothers. This is why I cried for him and why I missed him very much. The sixth brother studied fisheries at a school in Nagasaki and found a job in a big fishing company catching salmon in the Sea of Okhotsk. As a result, only two brothers remained in Nagasaki. The eldest owned my father's main store and the fifth worked with my parents in the new store. I always found myself alone in our house when I came home from school. It was a lonely life, but it was good to be able to read books in a quiet room of my own. Not very far from our house there was a bookstore which rented books. There was also a city library near the Suwa Shrine, only a ten minute walk from our house. I was attracted to books. First, it was books of fairy tales, but gradually I was introduced to books for adults such as mystery books and novels. I also read journals and Japanese classics. Instead of playing with other children during my primary and middle school days, I used to spend my free time reading in my quiet room. I was a lonesome boy.

Snow is rare in Nagasaki, but I saw snow falling on the Sunday morning of December 10, 1931. It was the first snow of that winter. It was such a beautiful morning. I could not stay at home. I took a walk in the street. After a moment of hesitation I decided to visit Tetsuji Koyano, my classmate, at his home. Stepping on the snow-covered street was exciting. I arrived at his home before long, but he was not at home. I was told that he went to Sunday School in a church behind his house. My curiosity led me to the church.

It was not a big cathedral like Urakami Catholic Church. It was a small wooden building. At the entrance I saw the name of the church, "Umamachi Congregational Church." As I tried to see inside, my eyes met those of the Sunday School children staring back at me, a stranger. Before I turned away, the familiar voice of Koyano caught my ear, "Why don't you come in, Kawano?"

I had no choice but to go into the small church. This was the first time in my life I had ever attended a church. I was only a young middle school student, a boy only thirteen years old. The Sunday School did not last long after I entered the church. Soon the Sunday morning service for adults began. Hymns were sung and a sermon read. I do not remember what the preacher told us, but I remember clearly the attractive atmosphere of the church. It was quite different from my dark, gloomy home. Not only the building but also the people, adults as well as children, looked happy and were smiling. The thought of approaching Christmas might have made them happier. To my surprise, I was assigned a role in a Christmas pageant. I joined the rehearsal with excitement, because I loved novels and dramas. It was my first Christmas. The play went well, as did my performance, which made me a little proud. I was accepted as a member of the Sunday School and welcomed to the church for the first time in my life.

Tetsuji was not my only acquaintance in the church. I found Mr. Masayoshi Chiba, a senior member of the volleyball team at Nagasaki Middle School, the same school I attended. I loved him and respected him because he was a gentle senior who encouraged us juniors in the volleyball court with a smile and humor. He was ready to run for the ball if it went outside the court, instead of commanding us to pick it up. I learned something new about him that Sunday, something I did not know before. I learned that the pastor of this church was his father.

Rev. Chiba was born in Kumamoto Prefecture. He had studied theology in Doshisha University, and had been the pastor of several churches before coming to Nagasaki. He was an honest and stoic old man, a typical Japanese of the Meiji Era (1868-1912). Mrs. Chiba was quite different. She always welcomed me with a warm smile as if she were my own mother. It did not take long before I felt more at home in the parsonage than in my own home.

I visited the church often, not only on Sunday but also on other days of the week. It became my new routine to visit the parsonage as soon as I came home from school. Mrs. Chiba welcomed me anytime. She prepared something sweet for us at tea time. Masakuni, an older brother of Masayoshi, stayed at home during the day and rested in bed most of the time because he had pulmonary tuberculosis. He was slim but looked healthy, with a handsome profile like that of a Greek god. He played the violin marvelously well and conducted the singing of hymns in church. He was an artist, a thinker, and a good reader. He had read many classics. He was also interested in theological and philosophical books. It was not long before the young boys and girls of the church adored him. A Young Men's Society was formed with Masakuni-san (san is a term of respect added to a man or woman's name, equivalent to Mr., Ms., or Mrs.) as the leader. My old friends Muneo Araki and Eiji Hirano joined the group. With other young boys and girls we studied the Bible and played together. Masakuni-san, who had experienced conversion at the age of twenty-three, was our leader, consultant and a good interpreter of the Bible.

In 1933, I was baptized without telling my parents, shortly after I had finished reading the book *Quo Vadis* by Sienkiewicz and was deeply moved by the hero, who kept his faith under the merciless persecution of the Emperor Nero. When my father, a devout Buddhist, learned of my baptism later, he was furious. He felt that it was a disgrace, not only for him but also for his ancestors, to have a heathen in his home. He could not live in the same house with a believer in a once forbidden foreign faith, and asked me to leave his Buddhist home unless I gave up my Christian faith. I stayed in the house without arguing with my father, waiting for the time when he would understand me.

I started to read the Bible alone. The first chapter of St. Matthew did not impress me at all but the story of Jesus' birth was interesting. The fifth chapter, "The Sermon on the Mount," caught my heart and soul. The words "Love your enemy" surprised me. I could have agreed if it had said "Love your parents and brothers," but what a contradiction to love an enemy we are supposed to hate and kill! How can a person like me who does not love his own mother be able to love an enemy? It is impossible.

My mother had no education. I was ashamed of her illiteracy. She was born in 1872 in the same village where my father was born a few years later. There was no primary school in a poor fishing village in those early days of the Meiji Era. Besides, education was regarded as unnecessary for a girl. My mother had to work hard in her youth and much harder after she was married to my father and raised seven boys one after another in Nagasaki. I was her last son. She expected a girl after six boys, but I disappointed her. She was already 46 years old and could not feed me at her breast. Every day I sucked the rich milk of a neighbor woman who had had her baby in the same month as my mother. As a result, I did not miss my mother. I had little affection for my mother and did not ask for her love, either. She worked and stayed in her workplace most of the time. I saw her only at mealtimes and in bed. She was too busy to be with her seventh son, leaving me to be taken care of by a maid or someone in the house. I was not very close to my mother.

Although I did not hate her, I did not love her. I was cold to her, or indifferent. Now, as a new convert to Christianity, I must love my mother, because Jesus ordered me to love everyone, including my enemy. If I could not love my mother, I should at least act as if I loved her. First, I decided not to blame her for everything. I said "It's good" when my brother complained about the food she prepared. I started to help her, after neglecting her for a long time. I stopped arguing with her and gave her warm words of appreciation instead. The result was surprising. The attitude of my mother changed obviously. She cared about me. She wanted to give me all the best. She saved for me rare delicacies, hiding them from the eyes of my brothers. I appreciated her caring for me and the affection that grew between us. The change convinced me that it is not impossible to love my enemy.

It is the enmity of mankind that invites human calamity. War will never happen if we overcome our enmity. It is contradictory that those who shout for peace blame each other and hate each other, because the enemy of peace is human hatred and enmity. It is an illusion to expect that the peace of the world can be established as soon as nuclear weapons are abolished. Peace can be maintained by abolishing enmity on both sides, not by blaming the defense forces and nuclear weapons of each side. Jesus ordered us to "judge not." That is the starting point of reconciliation between people as well as nations. This truth was revealed to me after I behaved as if I loved my mother. "Love your enemy" means to forgive others, whoever they are. It means to "hate the sin, but not the man," as a Japanese proverb said. It is the beginning and the end of love to treat others with good will and a warm heart even if we do not like the person. I found this truth at last.

I did not study at all until I entered middle school. Primary school teachers gave me "A" in all subjects, even though I neglected school work and read other books which attracted me more than the text books. I received "B" only once, and that was because of my behaviour in class. My teacher found me indulging in a novel rather than paying attention to the subject being taught in the classrooom. Nevertheless, I had been in the top of my class throughout my primary school years. On the day of graduation, I had the honor of representing all the new graduates by reading my gratitude speech to the school.

Before I became involved in the church I was not a good student. During my early days in middle school I did not like my teacher of mathematics, and I neglected to study mathematics. As a result, I was often scolded by the teacher. The more I was scolded, the more I hated the teacher and mathematics. I liked Japanese and Chinese classics because they were easier subjects for me. I was good at English because the teachers of English were good and I was curious about foreign languages. American movies might also have helped my progress in English. Although school children were not allowed to go to movie theaters, I dared to ignore the rule. Consequently I was regarded as a bad student who broke the rules of the school. My school record went down, as might be expected.

I changed, however, after I found the church. In addition, I met a good teacher to watch over me in my third year at Nagasaki Middle School. He was a tall, slim teacher named Mr. Tanaka. He was a teacher of mathematics but encouraged me by telling me that I should devote my time to the study of English, my favorite subject, instead of laboring in mathematics with little progress. When the time came to solve mathematical problems in class, Mr. Tanaka avoided calling my name. He always skipped me and asked the student in the next seat, who was better than I in mathematics, to answer the problem.

While I was struggling with a famous training book on English, *Good Interpretation of English* by Keijiro Ono, a model examination test was given to all fourth and fifth year students, equivalent to the 11th and 12th grades in the American system. I happened to be at the top among all the fourth year students. Mr. Tanaka was very pleased with the result. He praised me and encouraged me to try an entrance examination to Saga High School, one of three famous high schools in Kyushu. His reasoning was that I had a good chance in Saga High School because the test on mathematics counted only 50 points out of a total of 450, whereas the English language test was worth 200 points, and Japanese and Chinese classics were worth 100 points each.

My father had been against my entering the middle school. He permitted me to take the entrance examination only after my primary school teacher persuaded him that it was a waste of my ability to discontinue my education after primary school. I doubted, therefore, if my father would let me take the entrance examination to Saga High School. I knew that he would not oppose my going to the school of commerce in Nagasaki, which was located only ten minutes from our house. However, I could apply for the entrance examination of the school of commerce only at the end of my fifth year in middle school. I asked my father to let me try the examination at Saga in order to prepare me for next year's school of commerce test. He agreed, and I went to Saga to take the examination of Saga High School.

Actually, what I wanted was to be free in Saga. After taking the examination, I enjoyed the freedom of seeing European movies with no one behind me to watch over me. I did not care about the result of the examination. The competition was stiff and only one out of eleven applicants would be allowed to become a student of Saga High School. After coming back from Saga I went camping in the Nagasaki Peninsula with my friends and forgot about the test. When I came home from camping, I was shocked because people came one after another to congratulate me on my success. My father had to yield to the result of the examination. He agreed to pay the necessary expense for the school, but for only one year, no longer. It was in 1934.

# 35

# A TUTOR

"In this school you are gentlemen, We treat you as gentlemen from now on. Therefore, you must behave as gentlemen."

This is what Mr. Manji Ikoma, the Dean of Saga High School, announced to the new students on the first day of my high school year in 1934. It was a surprise for me, whose behavior had been restricted by the strict regulations of middle school. No one would give me orders any more. No one would keep an eye on me to find out my faults and law-breaking sins. To live as a gentleman is the only principle I must follow. What freedom! What a privilege! But what a great responsibility. I was exalted by this unprecedented treatment of a boy of sixteen. I imagine the young men of old-time Japan who reached the age of sixteen and had the ceremony of *genpuku* to signal the status of grown-up samurai must have experienced the same feeling of pride and responsibility. Karl Hilty wrote in his famous book *For Sleepless Nights* that love and good example are the secret of good education. I would add one more. It is faith, to trust one's students. And Dean Ikoma had the faith. One cannot expect a good result from education unless one trusts his students and reserves his criticism and interference. I hope the teachers today have the same love, good example and trust as Hilty and Dean Ikoma had.

The old Saga High School, which changed its name to Saga College after the war, was located in Honjo village in the suburbs of Saga city. The old wooden school building was built in 1920. The first year students were assigned to live in the adjoining dormitory. I shared a room with Nakao, who also came from Nagasaki MIddle School. I had no trouble with him, although once in a while I had to take care of him when he was drunk. I myself did not drink liquor. I had nothing to do with the "high school style" life with the torn kimono and dirty cap, wearing high wooden sandals and singing dormitory songs in a loud voice. Again, I found mathematics most disagreeable. No wonder, with my poor basic training, that I could not follow advanced mathematics. On the other hand, I enjoyed English lessons. They had a good staff of teachers in English. One of them, Professor Takahashi, was responsible for our class of 30 students majoring in humanistic arts. His textbook for us was Thomas Hardy's *Far from the Madding Crowd*. His nickname was "Gorilla" because of his short size and protruding mouth, but he was a kind person and often entertained us at his home. Professor Ishida was a contrast. He was a severe, intelligent gentleman with an ivory face and broad forehead. He taught us a mystery book by Conan Doyle. I could not wait for the end of the story, so I read the book ahead in haste, without taking time to look at the dictionary. When my name was called by the Professor, I had to come back to the page we were studying in the class and translate the sentence into Japanese. This method of reading through in a hurry must have improved the speed of my reading English. One loses interest if one has to read only one book in a year-long course of study. It would be much better to read it through in a short time, without stopping at every new word and digging into the dictionary each time. If you meet a new word many times in a book, you can grasp the meaning gradually and can limit the use of a dictionary to the key words you must know exactly. It was a pity that fast reading of English books had never been taught in schools in Japan. I developed the habit of reading other English books untaught at school. It made my study of English easier and enjoyable. This habit helped me later when I became fascinated by Agatha Christie and read her 65 books in two years.

The teacher of English conversation was an old, gray-haired gentleman from London. His English was polite and easy to understand. The King's English was taught in Japanese schools until the Second World War, and I had difficulty in getting used to American English later. On the other hand, it was to my advantage in Canada and Europe because people preferred British English to American English there.

Professor Ryuta Oda was a popular professor in Saga Higher School. He wore a Japanese kimono with *hakama*, or formal divided skirt, in school. His round face was covered with a gray beard. With his happy smile he led us to the world of Confucius. He gave us lectures in such an enthusiastic manner that we had no choice but to love the Chinese classics and the personality of Confucius. His nickname "Confucius" suited this beloved professor perfectly well. As a student interested in Chinese classics I attended his class faithfully, and repeated his course twice because I stayed in the second year class for two years for a reason I shall explain later. Therefore, I memorized the famous aphorisms of Confucius:

"Is it not delightful to have men of kindred spirit come to one from afar?"

"At fifteen I set my mind upon wisdom. At thirty I stood firm. At forty I was free from doubts. At fifty I understood the laws of Heaven. At seventy I could follow the desires of my heart without transgressing the right."

"When walking in a party of three, my teachers are always present. I can select the good qualities of the one and copy them."

"Is it not indeed a pleasure to acquire knowledge and constantly to exercise oneself therein?"

"The nobler type of man is broad-minded and not partisan. The inferior man is partisan and not broad-minded."

"Artful speech and an ingratiating demeanour rarely accompany virtue."

The school year starts in April in Japan and summer vacation begins in July. At the end of the first summer vacation, I came back to the dormitory before any one else returned. And I started to read a book I carried. It was *Uncle Tom's Cabin* by Mrs. Stowe. I was fascinated and read it through all night until next morning despite the attacks of mosquitoes. The impact of this book was great. I sympathized with Tom, a slave, who endured all hardship with faith and courage. I was impressed by Mrs. Stowe's humanity and her devotion to bringing freedom from slavery to America. Reading a good book in one's young days exerts a long-lasting influence.

During winter vacation in Nagasaki, my father told me, "We cannot afford to give you money for schooling any more. You must give up school by the end of March."

In the final semester, an English teacher called me and asked if I would work as a private tutor for a middle school boy. I thanked him for his help and accepted the offer.

The big house in which I tutored was the home of the biggest bookstore proprietor in Saga. My student was a twelve-year-old nephew of the owner, a son of his sister who had lost her husband and had come home with three children to work at her brother's bookstore. Sukehiro was the eldest son of Mrs. Mitsu Ito. He was in the first year of a middle school. To the disappointment of his mother, the level of his school work was found to be too low for him to be advanced to the second year class. So he needed a private tutor.

The Otsubo House was a big building. The owner was the eldest son of the founder, and his parents were still well and lived in the same house. Whenever I came home from school, this grandfather sitting in the living room offered me a cup of green tea. I thanked him and sipped the good green tea before I left for my room. This old gentleman, who had founded the bookstore and had success in his business, was also good in flower arrangement. Often I watched him arranging flowers in a beautiful porcelain vase. He understood and appreciated a traditional Japanese culture. I enjoyed being with him. I owe to him my love for Japanese tea and my interest in flowers and ceramic arts. I often saw his wife, the grandmother, in the garden where she took care of flowers and vegetables. She was also active in the kitchen, giving orders to the maids, and sometimes to her daughter-in-law, the mother of four children. At dinner time the table was crowded with seven children and their parents and grandparents. It was a big family, and all of them were nice to me because I was respected as a tutor, even though I was only seventeen.

As an inexperienced tutor I was often puzzled by my student, who ignored me. He answered in a low voice when I spoke to him, and hesitated to talk to me. I could not guess whether he disliked me or was merely awkward. Perhaps he was showing his determination not to study. I felt lost. What could I do if he did not want to study? I gave up. What I taught him first was how to play cards. After a time of hesitation, he started to play card games with me. But it was too late. By the time we became closer to each other, the first school year ended for him. The school told him that he had to start again from the beginning.I felt partly responsible for his failure, but Mrs. Ito admitted that it had been too late to look for a tutor near the end of the semester and politely asked me to stay with him so as not to deprive the boy of hope.

The busiest time for a bookstore is the spring, when the new school year begins. Otsubo Bookstore asked me to help in the store during the spring vacation and promised to provide me all my new textbooks free as a reward for my service. I agreed, and worked at the store, dealing with school children and students who rushed in for new textbooks. But it was a surprise to me when I learned that Mrs. Ito paid all my tuition for the second year in Saga High School. I thanked her for her kindness and promised to do my best for her eldest son.

# 36

# SURGERY

"Am I going to die?" I wondered in the darkness of a ward in the University Hospital, shortly after my second surgery.

I regret that I was careless after the first surgery. I was discharged from Tomonaga Hospital in Dejima within a week after an appendectomy, because there were not enough beds for the many patients who wanted to be operated on by Dr. Tomonaga, a famous surgeon in Nagasaki. I should have stayed longer in bed at home, but I went out on the next day and visited the middle school where I used to study, and saw students playing in the volleyball court. I was tempted to practise with them, and did so, but only for a brief time. Was this the reason why the small intestine herniated into the unhealed scar tissues under the skin? Or did it start when someone joked in the ward and I could not stop laughing in spite of pain in the operated area? I do not know. Not a single cause, perhaps. Anyway, I noticed that the surgical scar on the right lower abdomen swelled every time I stressed my belly. The diagnosis after examination was herniation in the scar. The skin surface healed well, but the tissues underneath were loose and weak. Abdominal pressure would easily cause herniation of the underlying intestine and swelling of the scar of the skin. It was possible that the herniated small intestine might develop inflammation and end in rupture and peritonitis. I was advised to have the second laparotomy to close the loose structures under the scar.

The second operation was performed in the University Hospital. I was carried to the surgical theater. A young nurse shaved my pubic hair with no hesitation, disregarding my blushing. Then I was asked to lie on my side. A long needle was injected into my spine and spinal anesthesia was given. I did not worry about the pain of surgery, because I had experienced no pain in the previous surgery. But as soon as the operation started, I felt intolerable pain.

I complained of pain, but the surgeons continued their work, paying little attention to my complaint. Professor Koyano ordered them to add local anesthesia, which reduced my pain but made me sleepy, and I lost consciousness for hours. It was in the darkness of a single room of the surgical ward that I found myself in the late evening. I was alone. No one was around. I was scared, by the darkness, by the loneliness, but more by the possibility of death.

I wanted to cry. This was not fair. I had had the luck of entering a high school, and had found new hope of continuing my study, thanks to my new post as a tutor. It was too soon to die at this young age of seventeen, without accomplishing anything in this world. I owe so much to so many people. I had learned much about life. I had been taught to dedicate myself to God and serve people. And yet I had done nothing by way of repayment for all I had received. A feeling of despair took over my heart. I sank in the darkness of my soul as dark as the room I was in. I prayed to God, asking forgiveness for my failure and uselessness.

The night was over. I was still alive. My room was filled with the bright sunshine of a spring morning. There appeared a nurse in a white uniform who asked me, "How do you feel this morning?" Her uniform shone in the sunlight and her warm smile radiated magnetic beauty. She was a real "angel in white uniform."

I did not die! My fear was groundless. God had given me another chance in life. How long? I did not know. But I knew that I could do something for Him. I could continue my study to prepare for the future. What a joy to have a life again in the new world! I must cherish my new life, for it was given to me anew from Him.

After discharge from the hospital I was more careful this time. My eldest brother advised me to rest in a hot spring spa called Michinoo in the suburbs of Nagasaki, and made the necessary arrangements for me. The day before I went to Michinoo I walked up to the Suwa Shrine Park to see the harbor of Nagasaki from my favorite place in the park. A large Torii gate of the shrine was only 100 meters from my house. A series of long stone steps led me to the shrine. Below the last long steps there was a stone-paved square where colorful shows and dances were dedicated to the shrine every October at the famous Suwa Festival. In my childhood I was eager to see the festival from the free seat of the stone steps, and went to the shrine before dawn to secure a seat. Memories of my childhood came back to me as I climbed the steps.

Suwa Park begins at the western end of the Shrine building. It is near the Suwa Forest where I used to play as a child. I found a familiar stone from which one can view Nagasaki's entire "Crane Harbor," shaped like the bird after which it is named. I saw ripples on the beautiful water and the deep blue color reflecting the May sky. The nearby park was filled with red and pink azalea flowers. I appreciated my happiness at being there. I wanted to share my happiness with someone.

One week in Michinoo Hot Spring Spa was also pleasant. This hot spring was only a few minutes' walk from Michinoo Station, the second station from Nagasaki. There were only a few hot spring inns. I stayed in a small one, next to a public bathhouse. I was introduced to the owner, Mr. Makita, and his family consisting of his wife and two children. There was also Mr. Makita's niece. Miss Tomoe Saito was seven years older than I, but we became good friends as soon as we found that we were both Christians. I was also introduced to her Christian friend, Miss Momoe Tomonaga, who happened to visit Miss Saito during my stay in Michinoo. We often walked to Michinoo Park and enjoyed discussing many subjects. They were both members of the Furumachi Church. I did not expect at that time that I would live in the Furumachi Church ten years later near the end of the war.

I came back to Saga with renewed strength and health. All members of the Otsubo family welcomed me. Sukehiro changed his attitude and studied obediently. I was eager to close the gap of my absence from school. My herniated scar gave me a good excuse to cease my club activity in *kendo*, Japanese fencing. But I became more active in the speech club and Bible study meetings. Professor Hideo Iwamoto was the adviser for the two groups. He was a son of a Buddhist priest but had studied philosophy in Kyoto University under the famous Christian Professor Seiichi Hatano, author of *The Origin of Christianity*. His doctoral thesis was a study of the Apostle Paul. He had a wide knowledge of Christianity as well as Buddhism. We had regular Bible study meetings. Our small group of Christian students met every week to study the Bible and discuss a variety of topics. It became my routine to read the Bible every morning and take note of key sentences.

When the summer vacation came again, I went on tour with our speech club and crossed the East China Sea. Our first destination was Dairen (Dalian), a major Japanese port city at the southern tip of Manchuria. The meeting was in a YMCA building. I gave a speech after other members. I do not remember what I said. All I remember is that I felt a sudden attack of pain in my lower abdomen when I finished my speech. All I could do was to step down from the stage. I was carried to my friend's home in Dairen. I knew the pain was caused by herniation inside the scar. I had to avoid any peritoneal pressure to the old scar. Lying in bed as quietly as possible was all I could do. The other members of the club had to leave for the next destination, Changchun. I stayed in the home of Matsuoka, my classmate born in Dairen. His family was kind to me. I felt at home and stayed for a month before I left for Saga alone.

I was admitted to a hospital in Saga and underwent further surgery. This time there was no pain during the surgery, and I never worried about death. All hospital expenses were paid by Mrs. Ito. I did not know how to thank her for her help to this young tutor. The Otsubo family treated me as if I were one of their family members. I felt deeply indebted. Of course I had done my best to help Sukehiro in his study.

To my satisfaction, Sukehiro improved his status in school. He finished the first year with good marks this time, and became a second year student at last. It was I who failed to pass the examination to be advanced to the third year class. The days of my attendance at school were insufficient to fill the requirement because of my repeated surgery that year. I was ashamed of my failure, and buried myself in the busy work of the bookstore in my third spring in Saga.

# 37

# THE BOARDING HOUSE

It was my first visit to Saga Prefectural Hospital. I went there to visit Miss Masako Tsuji, a member of the Saga Church. The hospital was located in the neighborhood of the Otsubo house where I lived. I looked for the tuberculosis ward, which was a separate building in the hospital because tuberculosis is a contagious disease. At the entrance, a nurse gave me a white mask to cover my mouth. In the corner of a room I found Masako lying on a bed.

"How are you, Masako-san?" I asked. She answered "Not so bad, thank you," with her fragile smile. Her face was as pale as white wax. I did not know her age, but she seemed several years older than I. She asked me in her quiet voice how I was doing.

"I had to remain in the same class for another year. I was admitted to hospitals three times and had surgery three times in one year. I was absent from school too long and missed many lectures. That was why I have to take the same course again. I hope I shall do better from now on. I am all right."

I observed the room while I was speaking to her. It was a gloomy room without any decoration or flowers. I expected to see someone in the room to take care of her, but no one was attending her in the room. I knew tuberculosis of the lung was contagious. People were afraid of contamination and avoided contact with patients.

"Even doctors do not see us often. Nurses come only when they have to. I miss my friends, but they don't come often. The room is quiet most of the time."

I thought her mother and sister would come to see her daily, but she said that they came only once or twice a week. I sympathized with her. It is cruel to leave a patient in solitude, even though the disease is contagious. It is surely the duty of a physician to visit his ward every day. I resented the neglect of the hospital staff. I sat down close to the bed and told Masako all the news about the church and my days in school and with the Otsubo family until a nurse came in and reminded me, "Don't stay too long. It is not good for the patient."

I knew that Masako was lonesome. Life in a hospital with a chronic disease is hard for anyone to endure, but Masako never complained. She listened to me in silence when I spoke to her of my experiences in surgery. Her eyes were fixed on mine and she kept her weak smile, but she made no complaint. She stayed there in bed like a statue of a noble, smiling girl, accepting and enduring all as fate.

On the way back from the hospital, I became angry. Everybody was unkind to tuberculosis patients, not only doctors and nurses but also their families. Christians are expected to visit sick people, but the attitude of the pastor of the Saga Church disappointed me. He had never visited Masako, even though he knew she had tuberculosis of the lung. He was concerned more about theology than the individual Christians in his church.

Jesus told the story of "The Good Samaritan" to his disciples because he wanted to teach them that the practice of love is more important than religious talk and ceremonies. A Jewish traveler was attacked by a robber on a road to Jericho. He was wounded and lying on the roadside in a shocked state. There came a Jewish priest who passed him without helping him. A Levite came, but he did nothing for the poor man. Then came a Samaritan, whom Jewish people disliked. He helped the man, took him to a roadside inn, asked the landlord to take care of him, and undertook to pay the landlord for all the care provided. Jesus was not a cynical man. He simply wanted to teach us the importance of love for another human being, the core of religion. He paid little attention to dogmatic controversies and religious ordinances. That was why he was despised and hated by the religious establishment and finally crucified on the cross.

Before he died, however, he prayed God to forgive those who had persecuted him and driven him to death because "they did not know what they were doing." I can see why a man shouted, "Look at him! He is the true son of the living God." I can understand that his disciples could not believe the death of their Master and developed their faith in his resurrection and his coming again. But I could not understand how a minister of the church of Christ could blame Masako for her absence in the Sunday service, and why he refused to visit her in the hospital.

She recovered gradually. Her temperature returned to normal. She wanted to rest in her own home, and her discharge was approved. I visited her at her house, often on the way home from church and from school. Then I thought that it would be much easier and more convenient to see her if I lived in her house as a boarder, because her mother rented her rooms to students and cooked for them.

It was quite a distance from the Otsubo house to Saga High School. I walked on foot to and from school, starting from the wide road lined with gingko trees, reaching the moat surrounding the old castle, passing by the Prefectural offices, and then coming to a large lotus pond. In cold winter it was covered with red leaves, but in spring large, round, green leaves came out, and then in summer the noble white lotus flowers attracted the eyes of passers-by. With the big old trees of the castle behind, it was a picturesque view. I enjoyed this daily walk to school, even though the sun scorched in summer and the cold wind made me tremble in winter. It was an enjoyable exercise.

In the early spring of 1937 I decided to resign my job of tutorship, not because the Otsubo house was far from school, nor because I had trouble with the Otsubo family. On the contrary, Sukehiro studied so well that he did not need a tutor any more. I felt guilty about staying in the house and receiving meals and all other expenses at school when I was no longer needed there. Besides, I wanted to have my privacy.

I asked Mrs. Ito permission to leave the house and told her of my intention to live alone in my last year of the high school. She was distressed and begged me to stay, but I assured her that Sukehiro did not need me any longer.

I made a temporary contract with the church. I was allowed to live in the attic of the church in exchange for my service of cleaning the church. But I had to eat something at least once a day. There was an old woman baking sweet potatoes for us students near the gate of the school. I was her customer. I negotiated with her and bought the privilege of eating as many potatoes as I wanted by paying her five yen a month. She was very kind. She knew that I would eat much more than I had paid for.

My father learned about my new situation and promised to send me the minimum sum of money I needed to support myself, at least for one year. At the same time I was told that a room was available in Masako's house, because a student had left. I did not miss the opportunity and moved to her house. It was located in a small alley not far from the school. My room on the second floor was small but quiet. I was satisfied with my new, private room as well as the meals prepared every morning and evening. Another boarder was a Korean student, who was a good young man to live with. I enjoyed having free time to read books. I visited Masako downstairs when I became tired of reading.

I read books at random. I wanted to read all books of good repute. It was in these days that Karl Hilty's *For Sleepless Nights* became my favorite book, which has never failed to give me good advice at every critical moment of my life so far. I also read books by Kanzo Uchimura, a unique Japanese Christian. Among those I read were his famous *The Greatest Heritage to Later Generations*, *Consolation for Christians*, and *How I Became a Christian*. All impressed me and had a lasting influence on me.

Japan went to war with China that summer. There were many students who believed in Marxism. Hot political and ideological arguments were common among students. I had to read books on social science and philosophy to prepare for discussion. The speech club members were usually argumentative. They discussed any subject, including Buddhism and Christianity and politics and war. At an open discussion in a public hall, I took up the problem of war between Japan and China and criticised the policy of Japan. I learned later that Professor Iwamoto was called to the police and had to apologize for my criticism of the Japanese army and the foreign policy of the Government.

It was already time for me to decide on my future. In my middle school days, my dream was to be a teacher of English or history in a women's high school, for I believed that the education of women was most important for the future of a nation.

My father had his own dream. He wanted me to study economics or law at Tokyo Imperial University and become a leader in politics or economics. It was not my choice. My interest shifted from English and history to the study of the Bible. I was tempted to study Greek, the basic language of the New Testament. Other targets were the history of Christianity and theology. The ideal place for my study was Doshisha University in Kyoto where two Chiba brothers were studying already. Masakuni-san told me that a scholarship would be available in the theological seminary if I had the recommendation of a pastor. Then I could study in Kyoto without my father's help. I wanted to get his approval.

I told Professor Iwamoto my intention of studying at Kyoto, where he studied many years ago. He told me, "It would be easier for your father to approve your study in Doshisha University if I asked him, because I am a Buddhist as he is." He took an opportunity of going to Nagasaki and visited my father in his home to tell him my plan and ask for his approval. I was not there, but the Professor told me later that he said to my father:

"Your son became a good Christian because he inherited your religiousness as a Buddhist. It is a fruit of your faith in a different way. Would you please forgive him and let him study what he wants to study?"

My father himself told me when I came home that he could not say "No" to the Professor who made the effort of coming to Nagasaki from Saga for his son. I promised in turn not to burden him financially for my study in Doshisha University, because the scholarship was available.

Masako was pleased by the news. Although she knew that she would miss me after my departure from Saga, she thought that after studying the Bible and theology I would become a good pastor.

In April, 1938, I left for Kyoto and started my study at the Theological Seminary of Doshisha University as one of thirteen new students of theology.

# 38

# THE BELL TOWER WITHOUT A BELL

Cherry blossoms were in full bloom in the yard of old Kyoto Imperial Palace. Flower petals flew in the air, blown by the soft spring wind, and fell on the kimonos of the girl students of Doshisha walking in the street between the Palace and Doshisha University.

The Theological Seminary building stood next to the big gate of Sokokuji, established in the fourteenth century as the headquarters temple of Rinzai Zen Buddhism. There was Amherst Hall in the west and the University Library on the other side of the street. One corner of the Theological building formed the shape of a bell tower. At the entrance of the building there was a staircase leading to a chapel on the second floor. One can climb to the tower from a side door of the chapel. I climbed up to the bell tower, but there was no bell in the tower. Even though I would not hear the sound of a bell, I would study the Bible and theology under this bell tower in the years to come. I had a happy anticipation. No plan was made yet for my future after graduation. The first thing I should do was to study hard. That was the main thing at this moment.

For the time being, I did not have to worry about food. Rev. Chiba and his family had moved to Kyoto from Nagasaki the previous year, and I was allowed to stay in the parsonage with the Chiba family and go to the school of theology from there. For me it was quite natural to be treated as a member of the Chiba family. I never thought of paying for the food. The parsonage was located in a quiet residential area in the northern section of Kyoto, and I learned later that Professor Yugawa, famous winner of a Nobel prize in physics, lived in the neighborhood.

Doshisha was founded by Jo Niijima. The Doshisha English School was opened in 1875 with eight students. They were joined in the next year by the "Kumamoto Band" of dedicated Christians from Kumamoto Prefecture, West Kyushu. This band was headed by Soho Tokutomi, who became later a nationally recognized journalist, historian, and social critic. The school grew steadily and finally became a university to "educate practical men of skill and conscience," but Niijima died of acute peritonitis on January 23, 1890, shortly before the university was opened. His influence lasted long in Doshisha.

Jo Niijima was born in 1843. He was a brilliant student of Rangaku, or Dutch studies, a new science originally brought to Japan in Dutch-language books and, after the 1850s, in English publications. At the age of 22 he secretly went aboard a ship at Hakodate harbor and left Japan, violating the Shogunate prohibition against overseas voyages by the Japanese people. After arriving in Boston, he found an opportunity to study at Amherst College with the help of the Hardy family. After graduating from Amherst College he studied theology at the Andover School of Theology. He was appointed as an interpreter for the Japanese delegation dispatched to the United States in 1871 under Tomomi Iwakura, Ambassador Plenipotentiary, and then accompanied him to Europe. Later he compiled a long report on education in the Western nations, providing valuable data and an outlook which contributed to the entirely new education system in the Meiji Era. He was asked by the Japanese Government to hold a key post in education, but he turned down the invitation. As soon as he graduated from the school of theology, he went to Kyoto to build a new school based on his faith. He died in Kyoto and was buried in Kyoto, his beloved city.

Among my twelve classmates there were four Koreans who had studied at a theological school in Korea but could not continue their study because the Japanese Government had closed the school. Other Japanese classmates had studied at Doshisha High School until they entered the theological seminary. Thus they were familiar with life in Kyoto. The only female student was Mrs. Katsuko Nomura.

Mrs. Nomura was a widow. She had graduated from Doshisha School for Women in 1929 and was married to a young scholar, Giichi Nomura, but he died young in 1937. She decided to study social work and Christian ethics following the recommendation of Professor Shigeru Nakashima, who had taught her late husband. She was living in Nishijin, the northern and oldest section of Kyoto, with her mother and her son Motoyuki. She was a frank, kind woman who often invited me for dinner at her house.

My disappointment came sooner than I had anticipated. Called from the financial office of the school, I went to the front desk of the office one morning. The clerk gave me a check for my scholarship but ordered me to give it back at the next desk. Though I had received the check, I was left without any money. The amount of the check was sufficient only for my tuition. No one had explained to me ahead of time that the scholarship meant free tuition and nothing more. I did not know that I had to earn money for my living. I felt cheated. I had to rely on the kindness of the Chiba family, who provided me with meals and a place to stay.

Lectures on the new subjects were interesting at first. The study of the Greek language was exciting, because it would let me read the New Testament in its original language, Koineh Greek, the colloquial Greek used widely in the first century of the Roman Empire. I carried Huddilton's textbook and memorized the vocabulary in the street car on my way to and from school.

Lectures on the New Testament by Professor Tominomori and on the history of Christianity by Professor Uoki were interesting and helpful. But the seminar on dogmatics by Professor A. disappointed me. The references were written in German and the other students could not read German well. The slow progress made me tired of the lectures. I skipped the class often. I admit that the Hitler-style mustache of the professor made me sick, too.

In summer he left for Italy with his Automobile Club students and visited Mussolini in Rome. After he came back to Kyoto he boasted about the welcome he had received from the fascist leaders. A professor of theology approving fascism! I could not respect him.

Professor Uoki advocated a new "Japanese Christianity." It was an age of fever. Even in Doshisha, a "Defense of Japan" club was formed, which harassed the theological students. The Japanese Army had occupied Nanjing and killed many Chinese including civilians, but China determined to continue her resistance to Japan. Japan was in the deep muddle of the endless war with China. The Tripartite Pact (1940) with Germany and Italy as three resourceless nations was a desperate attempt on the part of Japan to deal with a difficult if not hopeless situation.

According to the written rules of the school, military training was not a required subject for students of theology. I refused to attend the military training for that reason, insisting that "military training is not for theological students who study the Bible, which orders us not to kill."

The school manager called me to his office and begged me, "Please attend the military training, because otherwise the school might be closed by the pressure of the Army officers who are responsible for military training in this school." I replied, "I will attend the training if my absence would cause trouble for the school. But then you must change the rule, too." I remembered what I had seen in Kyoto Station several days earlier.

Mr. Fukushima was a senior student of theology. He was popular among the students and staff of the school. He was drafted from the school to the battlefield in China and was killed in battle. All the students of theology went to Kyoto Station when his cremated ashes arrived at the station. All of us bowed deeply to the white box held by a soldier with a black band of cloth around his arm. The box passed through our midst and disappeared in a car. A question arose in my mind.

Christ taught us, "*Love your enemy*." Why must a theological student who is a follower of Christ go to the battlefield and fight to kill enemies, breaking the commandment of Moses, "*Thou shalt not kill*"? Is it not against the teaching of the Bible for all the staff and students of theology to honor as a hero a student killed in the war? If we had to be drafted before or after our graduation and die like Mr. Fukushima in this war in China, all our study in the school of theology would be wasted. If a theology student cannot escape the national duty to serve as a soldier, it might be wiser to serve as a soldier first and study after the end of the service. I began to doubt the meaning of my study in Doshisha, where the theological staff seemed to be treating this war as a sacred war, under the influence of the Japanese Army and the nationalistic sentiment of the people.

At the end of September, Rev. Chiba was appointed as the pastor of Ohtou Church, and his family moved to the Western District of Kyoto. It was a new, larger church with a kindergarten. Masakuni-san and Masayoshi went to school on week days but were busy in church on Sunday. The church members were mostly women, including those who worked at the kindergarten. The atmosphere of the church was colorful and cheerful, and Masakuni-san was the center of attention among the young women. He had to take rests on account of his poor health, but he sang well, played the violin often, and spoke eloquently. He was also an idol in his house, well protected.

One day, after supper, I was chatting with Masayoshi at the table. Mrs. Chiba was cleaning the table. Then Masakuni-san barked at me, "Why don't you stand up and wash the dishes? You haven't paid a cent for your meal."

The words struck me. He was right. I should be ashamed of myself. In the home of a pastor whose income was modest, I stayed and ate without paying any money at all, as if I had the right to be supported. I was not their relative. They had no obligation to feed me free, yet I made no effort to help them financially. Shame on me. I should not stay.

On the next day, I moved to an apartment. My excuse was that I wanted to live alone and study more. No one stopped me. Pastors were rich in spirit, but poor in finance, particularly in wartime Japan.

I had no source of income. I asked the school to find work for me. The work I was given was to print a summary of the weekly lecture of a professor. With a stencil pen, I mimeographed the outline of Professor Setsuji Otsuka's lecture for the students in preparation for the next lecture. The subject of his lecture was systematic theology. Not only the radical dogmatics of Karl Barth and Emil Brunner, but also the new American theology of Reinhold Niebuhr were introduced to the student. It was a stimulating subject and I enjoyed working for Professor Otsuka. I could not attend his class because it was not in the first year program, and yet I absorbed Professor Otsuka's views. It enriched my thought, but not my poor wallet.

Often, with no money in my pocket, I had to live on water alone. Mrs. Nomura's occasional invitation was exactly like "meeting Buddha in the Inferno" (a Japanese expression for great joy when one is rescued from a disaster). But my pride did not allow me to let her know my financial problem.

To my relief, a room was offered me in the dormitory for theology students. I could eat in the dining room of the dormitory. Payment could be postponed if necessary. There was no cost for transportation, because the dormitory was next to the school. And I found it enjoyable to live and talk with other theology students in the dormitory.

The dormitory was an old, Western-style building, but we lived on tatami reed-mats, as in a Japanese house. The ceiling was very high and in winter the room could not be heated well with a poor Japanese charcoal heater. I had to experience the cold winter in Kyoto for the first time. It was too cold for anyone born in Kyushu, the South of Japan.

I caught a cold, and cough and sputum continued. Complaining of fatigue, I visited a clinic, and tuberculosis of the lung was diagnosed. Without hesitation, I submitted my resignation from the school, accepting my illness as a Providential gift. I did not consult with anyone, because I had no need of consultation. I had no longer the desire, the funds, and physical strength to continue my school life.

It was a relief that I was no longer obliged to attend military training in Doshisha against my will, but my privilege of postponing military duty as a student was lost, and I would be called for physical tests. But it was obvious that the Army would not take a man with tuberculosis. Even if I were drafted, I could start my study again after my survival of military service and the war. This was better, both for me and for Doshisha, because I did not want to jeopardize the theology school through my conscientious resistance to military training.

I left Kyoto for Nagasaki with no regret at all.

# 39

# RAINBOW BEACH

Dr. Takahara was a family physician in Nagasaki. His nickname was "Water-doc" because he ordered patients to drink more water rather than giving them many drugs and injections. He was a man of humor, and encouraged patients with his smile and jokes. In pre-war Japan the biggest cause of death was tuberculosis of the lung, due to tuberculosis bacilli and poor nutrition. For a poor patient, a doctor who treats tuberculosis with water without using expensive drugs was a savior. Tuberculosis had been regarded as an "incurable disease" until streptomycin was discovered. It was a waste of money to buy expensive "special drugs" or to expect healing from costly injections. The money should be spent for good food and bed-rest in the clean air.

No wonder that many tuberculosis patients in Nagasaki came to Dr.Takahara's clinic. Mild cases of tuberculosis were cured by the treatment of this "Water-doc," or healed spontaneously. His reputation went higher and higher. Advanced cases died, of course, but as a professor of Nagasaki Medical School once confessed to us, "I felt sick when a professor of internal medicine examined me, but I felt relieved and half-healed as soon as Dr. Takahara called my name at the door of my room."

His sunny, kind and gentle personality was a salvation for gloomy sufferers of illness. They found hope in him. They tried to eat more. They felt better and the whole family regained confidence. It was a natural, favorable consequence following a visit with Dr. Takahara. The term "psychosomatic medicine" was not yet known, but Dr. Takahara practised psychosomatic medicine already in Nagasaki.

He was a Buddhist who respected Shinran, the founder of the True Pure Land Sect of Mahayana Buddhism in the thirteenth century. In his school years in the First Higher School in Tokyo and in Tokyo Imperial University Medical School, he studied Buddhism under the guidance of Rev. Umehara. Dr. Takahara influenced many Buddhist students in Kyushu. One of them was Professor Yujiro Ikemi of Kyushu University, the first Professor of Psychosomatic Medicine in Japan, who often went to Nagasaki to learn from Dr. Takahara.

I visited Dr. Takahara as soon as I came back to Nagasaki from Kyoto. He assured me of a good recovery. I stayed on the second floor of my father's store. Day after day I rested in bed looking at the ceiling. I had nothing to do but keep waiting for the recovery of my damaged lung. My thoughts drifted but always came back to the ugly aspects of myself. I disliked myself. I nearly gave up. My selfishness, impoliteness, and all my other disgusting characteristics were inherited from my parents. They were inborn "karma" and impossible to change. It was not my fault. The blame was on my parents.

Suddenly there came into my mind an answer of Jesus to the question of his disciples in the ninth chapter of St. John's Gospel: "*Master, who did sin, this man or his parents, that he was born blind?*" "*Neither hath this man sinned, nor his parents: but that the works of God should be manifest in him.*"

At this moment I was elevated to a sunny blue sky beyond the dark ceiling of the room. Karma from the unknown past and the bondage of sin inside me were cut off and I felt the first complete freedom in my life. The rest of my life would be a manifestation of the works of God. I should not worry about myself. All I have to do is to serve God and mankind as much as I can.

The symptoms of my tuberculosis were mild and recovery was fast, because it was found in its early stage. After three months of rest at home, Dr. Takahara permitted me to leave my bed. My father suggested that I stay for a while on the north coast of Saga Prefecture in the clean environment of the beautiful seaside resort called "Niji no Matsubara," which means Rainbow Beach of Pine Trees. A room in a small Japanese inn at the foot of Mirror Hill was rented for me. From my room on the second floor I could see the famous Rainbow Beach with one million pine trees growing along the beach for a mile in the shape of a rainbow curve, a spectacular view.

I spent my whole morning reading. After lunch I took a walk to the beach. Each one of the countless pine trees had its own unique shape. Walking alone through the pine forest was a new, exciting experience for me. After walking toward the sea for a while, I suddenly caught a glimpse of the sea between the bent trunks of pine trees, followed by the whole view of the Sea of Genkai and the dazzling white sand of the beach. Walking on the warm, ankle-deep sand I approached the water and sat on the sand. A large wave swept in from the ocean toward me and dashed onto the sand, almost engulfing me. I jumped up and retreated to the dry sand on a higher slope. Sitting on the sand, I kept watching the waves coming in one after another. It was a grand view, including a glimpse of Karatsu City at the far west end of the bay. Here is no school of theology, no military training, no politics, no army and no public. Only nature, marvelous nature, unchanged for ages.

One day Hirano, my old pal, came from Nagasaki to see me. We had a wonderful time together enjoying this Rainbow Beach. On another day on the beach I met a pale woman who was also a patient with tuberculosis of the lung in the recovery stage. We had common subjects to talk about and became good friends. No other visitor or friend had I during my short summer at this Rainbow Beach.

My happy stay at the beach had to be ended, however, because I received an order from the Army to take a physical examination for military service as a result of my desertion from school.

I had expected to be dismissed after examination because of my recent illness of the lung and the obvious scar in the lung on the x-ray film. However, I was surprised. There was neither examination by a physician nor x-ray test of the lung. We were asked to stand in line totally stripped. The examining officer gave a glance at all of us and then announced, "You have all passed the examination and are adopted as new soldiers, every one of you, with no exception." I was appalled, and then disappointed.

In May of this year, 1939, a dispute over the northwestern border of Manchuria and the People's Republic of Mongolia in the vicinity of Nomonhan led to a major conflict between the Japanese Army and the armies of Mongolia and the USSR. The confrontation ended in the unexpected defeat of the Japanese Army in August.

This "Nomonhan Incident" was not reported in Japan, and we did not know about this sad result of the conflict. Irritated by the prolonged war between China and Japan, and faced by the great menace of Russian Power, the Japanese Army leaders decided to reinforce the Guandong Division of the Army and recruited millions of new soldiers to get ready for a possible Russo-Japanese war. The Army needed every one of the Japanese youth and intended to give hard training to those "meek" fellows like me.

I expressed my wish to serve in the Medical Corps under the banner of the Red Cross to help the wounded and the sick, instead of killing other human beings. But the last report I received assigned me to an artillery unit and ordered me to report to the Artillery Regiment in Kurume, Kyushu, in February, 1940.

I did not want to waste the six months I had before going into the army. I went to Kyoto and asked at Doshisha for permission to attend Professor Hatano's seminar on the history of religion. I had plenty of time to read books. One book impressed me the most and inspired my choice of a career. That book was *Out of My Life and Thought* by Dr.Albert Schweitzer, translated into Japanese by Michio Takeyama and published in February, 1937, six years after Dr. Schweitzer wrote its last sentence in 1931. His name was unknown in Japan when I read this book. It was much later that Kanzo Uchimura introduced him in his journal of Bible study and sent Dr. Schweitzer the collected donations of his readers.

Dr. Schweitzer was born in Alsace in 1875 and studied theology at Strasbourg University. He was an organist, too. His pipe-organ recording of Bach's choral is one of my favorite musical records. On his 30th birthday, this outstanding theologian pipe-organist decided to become a doctor for the people of Africa. His motivation was a pamphlet from the Missionary Society in Paris he read in 1904. In an article entitled "What is Lacking in Missionaries in the Congo," Alfred Begner, an Alsatian, pleaded for the need for talented missionaries to go to northern Gabon. He wrote: "The Church is looking for a man who will respond to the call of our Lord and say, 'Yes, I shall follow thee.'"

This one sentence struck Dr. Schweitzer and motivated him to study medicine. He realized that he was suited more to the practice of love than the preaching of love. He decided to dedicate himself as a missionary doctor working for black Africans.

"All my relatives were against my plan, which seemed foolish," but he started the study of medicine in October, 1905 at Strasbourg University, where he continued his lectures in theology. Every Sunday he preached at the St. Nicolai Church as before. And also he founded the Bach Society in Paris and often gave organ recitals. It was a superhuman activity, "an endless fight against fatigue," as he decribed it.

His medical studies were finished in December, 1911. He passed all his examinations. Fund-raising took one more year. Finally he left Bordeaux for Africa on the 26th of March, 1913 with 70 crates of materials to build a hospital for the people in Lambarene, French Equatorial Africa, now called Gabon.

He dedicated the rest of his life to his "black brothers," as a living example of his philosophy of "reverence for life" until he died in 1965 some months after his 90th birthday. The hardships and sufferings he experienced in his half-century of life in Lambarene were described in his book. But what attracted me most was his principles of life:

"Only the man who can find meaning in every task and devote himself with full responsibility deserves an unusual mission. Only the man who knows how to carry out his duty with cool determination instead of heroism can be a spiritual adventurer in a society. There is no hero of action, but a hero of patience and self-renunciation."(p. 128)

"In all situations, a man works for another man with true human spirit ....here lies the future of mankind."(p. 131)

When I came to this sentence in the train for Tokyo, I left the train at the next station, walked to the beach and sat down on a stone. I was overwhelmed by a strong desire to study medicine in order to serve sick people as Dr. Schweitzer did in Africa.

At the end of January, 1940 I went to the Rainbow Beach again to say farewell to the view of Karatsu Bay and the rough waters of Genkai. The midwinter view of the beach was entirely different from what I saw in summer. From the nearest train station I walked under the dark, cold clouds to an old beach hotel. The maid in the hotel looked at me suspiciously, because it was not the season for swimming. She led me to an empty room. There was no other guest in the hotel. When she opened the closed window halfway, a cold wind struck the window. I saw big waves rushing toward the beach tossing up white foam. After my room service supper, no one dared to approach this lonely guest. I went to bed early and meditated on my past and unknown future.

I was a lucky boy. I was the only one in my family who was allowed to go to high school and university, while the other six brothers did not have the opportunity. But my special privilege was that I had found Christ, and this had led to many good friends and teachers, directly or through books.

My dream of studying in Doshisha was interrupted. Life in Kyoto was hard and I developed tuberculosis of the lung. It was cured faster than I had expected, but the duty of army service was waiting for me. The Sino-Japanese War seemed endless, and the ashes of soldiers killed in battle were coming home every day from the continent. Some day I might end up in a white box like the one I saw at Kyoto Station. Even if I did not die on the battlefield, my lung disease might recur and kill me in an army hospital. This evening might be my last chance to see the Sea at Karatsu Bay and listen to the sound of the wind coming through Rainbow Beach. The future is unknown, all is in the hand of the Almighty.

When night came, snow started to fall and started to blow, making a loud noise on the closed window. The wind blew harder and harder at midnight. The sound of waves became louder and louder. The stormy night of Rainbow Beach lasted long. I could hardly sleep.

# 40

# THE BLUE DRAGON

I reported to the 24th Artillery Regiment in Kurume on the fourth of February. New army uniforms and heavy fur coats were given to us. Two days later the new soldiers were sent to Moji Port by train, and put into a big freighter which left Japan and headed north. I thought we were going to China, but instead of landing in China, we disembarked at Rajin (Najin), a port on the northeast coast of Korea, followed by a long train trip to the north. It was the coldest winter I have ever experienced. I ate a frozen orange for the first time in my life. Our long journey from Japan ended on the border between the USSR and Manchukuo. The name of this land was Daijoshi (Dachengzi), an isolated region of the Mudanjiang District.

It was a barren land. There was no tree standing. No mountain was in sight. In the north, there was a group of buildings on a low hill. We were told that they were stables. Beyond the stables we saw nothing but a wide, hilly skyline. We learned later that Russian guns were ready to shoot us at any time from the tochka, pillboxes, built and hidden on the border.

As the new soldiers of the 212th Japanese Division in Manchuria, we had no time to look at the wild view, no time to be sentimental. A busy schedule from 5 a.m. till 9 p.m. started immediately, leaving no spare time for ourselves. The only time I found to read my tiny New Testament was a few minutes in the toilet.

It was nearly -40°C in the early morning when we were driven out of our bed to run uphill toward the stables. We had to carry the soiled, heavy straw out of the stable and spread it on the open ground. I stumbled often while I was running, and my hands easily slipped from the heavy bars of the stretcher. Each time came the shout, "Don't stop!" or "Hold the bars tight!"

After carrying out the wet, soiled straw, we began brushing the horses. Holding the bent leg of a horse, one must dig out the dirty stuff inside the hoof with an iron tool, before painting the hoof surface with oil. I was scared when a horse suddenly turned his long head toward me and glared at me. I hesitated to hold his leg, which might kick me any time. A senior soldier taught me to give a friendly pat on the back of the horse before approaching the leg. He demonstrated how to do it. The horse was used to him, but not to us beginners. He looked at me with suspicious eyes when I timidly touched his back. He pulled away his leg when I fearfully picked up his foot.

It took more than a week to master the technique of hoof cleaning. On the other hand, brushing the horse's fur coat was rather enjoyable after finishing the hoof cleaning. The horses liked the brushing. They stood still with their eyes closed or blinking, occasionally swinging their tails with obvious satisfaction. It was the time when horse-human relationships could be improved.

I did not expect horses to pull our field guns, because I thought tractors would do this job. In this regiment, however, they used horses instead of tractors. We were horsemen rather than soldiers. Riding horses was another new experience for me. I was not so reluctant to take riding lessons as to clean the stables. Under the wide, clear blue sky, the horse galloped under my feet on the endless plain of wild grasses. I had to hold the rein tightly to keep from falling out of the uncomfortable saddle. Nevertheless, it was a time of relief, a rare freedom in the dungeon life of a low-rank soldier.

The hardest work was the work in the stable. Every morning we had to run to the stable and carry out the heavy, soiled straw and spread it on the open field to dry until evening. My hands became numb sometimes, my arms ached often, and my legs stumbled every time. The hard labor was repeated every morning and every evening except Sunday, in the coldest winter as in the hottest summer. I was not sure how long my frail body, recently recovered from tuberculosis, could tolerate this hard life.

For the newcomers there were many extra tasks. The preparation of the meal table and the cleaning of dishes were also our duty. We were chagrined because the rice in our bowls was supposed to be less than in the bowls of older men who did not prepare meals and did not work as hard as we did. And I was the slowest in eating meals among the miserable new soldiers. Before finishing my meal I had to run out of the room with the other boys to clean the table and dishes. After such hard labor I could not satisfy my hunger, although other smart fellows quickly ate the food left on the plates before cleaning them in the cold outdoor kitchen with their chapped hands.

During my first three months in the army I lost weight, dropping from 57 to 52 kilograms. There was no doubt that my lung tuberculosis would recur sooner or later and I would be sent to an army hospital, then home. But my expectation was wrong. I survived the hard life, partly because the indoor environment in the Manchurian regiment was not so bad as the outdoor one. The brick building of the regiment was windproof, and warmed efficiently by the Russian-style brick stove called pechka. The outdoor temperature went down as low as -40°C but the air was not humid and snow fell rarely. The amount of rice in the meals was not much, but the food was rich in beans and pork. More and more unpolished millet and kaoliang grains were added to the rice, as the shortage of rice progressed. As a whole, nutrition was better than in Japan.

My crisis was avoided by the change of my role from a horseman to a gunner. I was assigned to clean the field guns rather than the horses. There were not many new soldiers who had higher education. Most of them were farmers or blue collar workers. Intelligence and technology were required for gunners. Each field gun needed five gunners, 20 men in the whole of our First Company, with four field guns.

The newly assigned gunners ran to the garage every morning, and polished the big guns and checked them to keep them ready for use. No perspiring work at all. The field guns were always clean, without a smear or smell of horse manure or urine. They did not actually need much work to clean them. All we had to do was to remove dust from the surface and to inject oil into the joints. The ranking private, or lance corporal, named Maeda was a quiet man from Arita, a town in western Saga Prefecture famous for its porcelain. He treated us with fairness. He kept his eyes on the stables in the distance. As soon as he saw the work in the stable coming to an end, he ordered us to stop working. After a quick line-up, we ran a good distance to our regiment building under the command of Superior Private Maeda, with less fatigue and less hunger than I experienced in the stable.

When the day of the grand autumn maneuver approached, shooting training began for us. It was training for readiness, adaptability and accuracy in shooting. I was the second gunner of the first platoon. My job was to regulate the angle of the gun and the scale of distance as quickly as possible according to the changing figures reported by the measuring team. My job was to aim at the target with perfect accuracy and quick response. The main reason why I was assigned to this key post of a field gun was my good eyesight: 2.0 in each eye. I thanked my parents who gave me good visual accuracy. My good eyesight also helped me win the top medal at a rifle shooting contest before the maneuver. The grand annual maneuver of the 212th Regiment was held on a beautiful autumn day. It was a big shooting contest of 16 companies in four battalions, and we belonged to the First Platoon of the First Company of the First Battalion.

Each of the four field guns of the First Company was pulled to a low hill by six powerful horses. Four hundred meters ahead of us, there was a white concrete tochka with a 30 x 100 cm window. It was our target.

I corrected the aiming scale quickly whenever a new report came from the measuring team.

"Now, shoot!", shouted the platoon leader. The gun was fired, and a shell of 65 millimeters in diameter flew toward the tochka. A spray of sand jumped behind the tochka, but a referee shouted, "No track of the shell."

The second shooting ended with the same result. We fired the third, and the last. Then a soldier ran to the tochka and checked the mound of sand behind the tochka. After a few seconds he screamed, "Hit! All three hit the target!"

The open window of the tochka was intact when the first shell and the second shell ran through the center of the window. Only the third one touched the rim of the window slightly and made a noise. All three shells were found deep in the mound of sand behind the tochka through which they had penetrated into the sand.

Our field gun among all the guns in our battalion was the only gun which hit the target three times. The achievement of our platoon was the best in the regiment. As the best gunner in the regiment, I was awarded a medal by the commander of the regiment. At the end of my first year in the army I was promoted from second class to first class private.

A group of fresh soldiers arrived in 1941 from Japan. We upper-ranking privates were relieved of our duty on meals. The volume of our rice increased, though not as much as that of the third-year soldiers. Our position between the newcomers and the third-year group was delicate. When we were the newcomers, the second-year group punished us at night for every minor fault. I used to tell myself "I would never do the same foolish thing with new soldiers." I kept my word, and did not punish my younger soldiers. It was my fellow second-year privates who complained,

"Why don't you allow us to hit the new privates? After all, we endured the punishment of the older soldiers, thinking of our chance in the next year to punish the new ones."

"I do not hit them because it was a bad tradition to torment the newcomers. We are responsible for the training of younger soldiers. If anything is wrong with them, it is our fault. Why don't you hit me, the head of the second-year soldiers," I used to reply, and they grumbled. The third-year soldiers were more difficult to handle. They told me, "The soldiers must be trained with fists. If you don't hit them we shall hit them."

I decided not to let them hit the fresh ones. After calling them all together one night, I announced, "I don't want our seniors to touch you. I would rather hit you with my fist than have you get beaten by senior soldiers. Forgive me." And I gave a heavy blow on the cheek of every new soldier, one after another, with tears falling from my eyes. Every young one stepped forward to receive my fist. I saw tears in some eyes. I did not know whether they were tears of anger or of compassion.

I was not yet free from fist blows. There was a corporal named Ishimaru, who marked me as an "anti-militarist." He knew the report on my behaviour in Doshisha, openly denouncing the military training in the school. He knew why I was not promoted to the rank of lieutenant like the other comrades who had attended military training at school. I had to salute them now as a private soldier.

Corporal Ishimaru was a professional soldier born in Saga Prefecture and an expert in handling horses. He looked great when he was riding on a horse. He had a powerful build and powerful arms. His fist hit me often for minor reasons, sometimes with no good reason, because he hated any anti-military intellectual. Once he started to hit me with repeated heavy blows of his fist. I did not beg his pardon, because I found no reason to apologize to him. The blows continued a hundred times before he gave up. One side of my face turned blue and I could not eat anything on the next day due to severe swelling of the left eyelid, cheek and mouth. It was a terrible experience.

There were a number of horses in our company. My favorite horse was a bluish gray horse with many white spots. His name "Seiryuu" means "blue dragon" in Japanese, a mysterious imaginary creature flying in and on a cloud. He had a quick temper. His sharp eyes stared at me when I approached him. Keeping his head high above the other horses, he trampled the floor of the stable. He was restless, hardly accustomed to life as a prisoner in this remote end of the earth. His proud, lonely figure had a strange charm for me. I even felt friendship for him, or empathy between us. Often on my free day, I visited this blue dragon. Tenderly touching his neck, I imagined the figure of Seiryuu running alone on a wild hill in the blue light of the moon at midnight. I understood the restlessness of Seiryuu, who wanted to cut off all the binding ropes and run away into the free world. I wished I could free him and run with him out of this imprisonment into freedom.

One day in my second year in the army, I was sitting next to Corporal Hayashi during a short rest period between field trainings. He looked at me and asked, "Kawano, you must be used to the army life by now. What do you think of our life in the army?"

"Lack of freedom is the hardest thing for me," I answered. He was surprised.

"Lack of freedom? Why? Don't we have a lot of freedom?"

I was surprised, too. So there must be plenty of freedom for a low-ranking, non-commissioned officer in this isolated regiment. He had to serve someone in civilian society, but as a corporal in the army he has unbridled power over his subordinate soldiers, who are not allowed to resist him. Even the captain, a graduate of the Military Academy, and lieutenants, graduates from other colleges, did not interfere with the action of these NCOs who were free to use their almighty power over the private soldiers. That was why no one stopped Corporal Ishimaru's harsh beating of me.

I must admit, however, that there were also kind NCOs who cared for and protected me. Mr. Ichiji Nakamura, a master sergeant, was one of them. He did not protest openly against the conduct of Corporal Ishimaru, but he sympathized with me, and called me often to help him with his paper work. I knew his intention. He wanted to put me under his care and he made others know that he needed me or was behind me. I appreciated his consideration.

Another good man was Mr. Kihachiro Yamasaki, a warrant officer. He liked to joke and he laughed in a happy way. It was he who recommended me as a desk clerk in the commendation office of the regiment. Every day, as soon as I had finished breakfast, I went to the commendation office room located in the center of the regiment, and worked at my desk. Most of my work was to write official documents in correct and decent Japanese. Our office staff consisted of a small group of officers and clerks. All were well educated people with skill in beautiful handwriting, both with the split-point pen and the *fude*, the supple writing brush. Working with them daily for the rest of my days in the army was very helpful to improve my brush-writing of Chinese characters and the Japanese syllabary.

The commendation office provided me with information which was secret from ordinary soldiers. It was in this office that I learned of the "Nomonhan Incident." I learned also about the "Kantokuen," a secret plan of the Japanese Guandong Army in Manchuria to occupy the USSR's Far Eastern territory following Hitler's attack on the Soviet Union in June, 1941. For this purpose 700,000 troops, 140,000 horses and 600 aircraft had been concentrated in northern Manchuria by August, 1941, but the highest authorities in Tokyo decided not to attack the Soviet Far East if the USSR would observe their Neutrality Pact with Japan of April, 1941and refrain from making attacks on Japan. Not being able to determine whether Germany could defeat the Soviet Union and enable Japan to pursue its original plans against the Soviet Union, the Japanese government decided to advance southward in the Pacific and Southeast Asia against what it perceived to be a four-power encirclement of Japan by the ABCD powers: America, the British, the Chinese, and the Dutch. Thus, on December 8, before Japan's declaration of war could be presented to the American president, the Japanese attacked Pearl Harbor and promptly mounted attacks against the British and the Dutch in Southeast Asia.

# 41

# A NEW MEDICAL STUDENT

In 1942 a new commander came to our company. He was Captain Fumio Yugawa. One day I was ordered to come to his office. It was a few days after I had told our cadet leader of my desire to work as a medical orderly in the regiment. As soon as I entered the room, he asked me, "Why do you want to be a medical orderly?"

"I am a Christian, Sir. I am not allowed to kill another human being. I like to take care of sick people, and I believe this kind of work agrees with my faith."

"As a citizen of the Japanese Empire, which order do you follow first, the Emperor's or Christ's ?"

"I don't think the Emperor would order me to do anything against the teaching of Christ."

Captain Yugawa was obviously displeased with my answer. He examined me in silence and then announced, "You may leave, now."

I could not guess how Captain Yugawa felt about my answer, but nothing happened afterward. My wish was ignored and I stayed as a gunner. I hoped that I would never be sent to the battlefront where people had no choice but to kill each other.

In April, a new army surgeon was assigned to our regiment. He was Dr. Nonaka, a graduate of Nagasaki Medical School. As soon as I heard about him, I visited him in his office.

"I have applied to be a medical orderly, but my application was not approved because I have no experience in medical care. Now I am considering the study of medicine after my discharge from the army. Is there any possibility of my acceptance in a medical school, even though I took the liberal arts course in high school instead of science?"

"Of course there is. If you pass an examination to test your aptitude for the medical course, you can apply for the entrance examination to the medical school. It will not be too difficult now as the shortage of doctors is so serious."

Encouraged by his words, I made up my mind to apply for the medical school examination. Dr. Nonaka kindly lent me books which were needed for my preparation. I devoted all my spare time to the study of mathematics and science.

Fortunately I was already a third-year soldier promoted to the rank of Superior Private, free from minor duties and manual work. I had my own time to use freely for study. No petty officer or corporal would torment me now. No hungry stomach any more. No one checked my mail or sneaked my package. On the contrary, younger soldiers presented me a share of their delicious gifts from home. My body weight increased to 64 kilograms, a new record for me.

We often anticipated the time of our discharge from the army, but were disappointed each time. I thought of helping and serving my mother after my homecoming. Since I came to the army and experienced the hard labor of new private soldiers, I sympathized with my mother who had worked for my father and for us seven children 70 years of her life. Now I had learned how to wash and cook. When I got home again, I would tell her how much I appreciated her service to us, and I would do all I could for my mother.

At the end of my third year, I was promoted to Lance Corporal, the highest rank for a private. A few days later, I received a sad letter from my father.

"Your mother died on the 3rd of February. I hesitated to tell you about her illness, because I did not want you to worry about her. She caught a cold in this cold winter and developed pneumonia. High fever continued, but she kept saying that she wanted to see you. She begged us to take her to Manchuria to see you before she died. Death came so suddenly that we cannot believe it even now." Holding this letter, I went outdoors and wept in the freezing cold air under the star-spangled sky of Manchuria.

In April, 1943, I came back to Nagasaki after three years and two months of army life. The city of Nagasaki had not changed much during my absence, but my father had. He was no longer the tough, active father I remembered. He was now a tired, lonely old man with gray hair who welcomed me with tears in his eyes.

He was no longer active in his business. Flour, sugar, and many other materials necessary for cake making were no longer available. They were all under the wartime control of the government. They lasted for only a few days a month. His shop had to be closed the rest of the time. The main store, which my father had given to my eldest brother, was already sold off to pay the large debt accumulated by my brother's gambling life. My brother had slipped away to Nanjing, China, where he opened a shop and occasionally sent money to his father, though barely enough to support him.

I could not see my father without sympathy. He was so glad about my return from Manchuria that he wanted to do everything for me. He was a born hard worker. He worked and worked to fight against poverty. He brought up seven boys, but no one was staying at home now. Near the end of his life he had suddenly lost his faithful wife, and now he was left alone in the empty house. I was glad that I had come back to him, two months after the death of my mother.

The entrance examination for medical school was not given for several months. I looked for a temporary job and fortunately found one in the conscription office of the Nagasaki Regiment, not very far from our house. My career in the army and my new title of corporal, which I received on the day before my discharge, were good recommendations for me. My work was simple. I wrote addresses on envelopes every day. Once a week I had a chance to practise *kendo* with my colleagues.

Nagasaki Medical School was in the Urakami district of the city. One day I went to the Medical School to present my application papers for the entrance examination. Then I visited the Department of Radiology and asked for radiographic examination of my lung. When my x-ray film came out, Associate Professor Nagai checked the film and said to me, "There is a trace of recurred tuberculosis in this film, but it is not active now."

When he learned that I had been in the army service until a few months ago, he told me in a brisk, clear-cut army accent that he had also returned only recently from his medical service in Southern China.

One month later I took the entrance examination without confidence, because I knew I was not good in physics, chemistry and mathematics. The result was unbelievable. I received a report telling me that I had passed the examination. I suppose that there were not many students who wanted to study medicine at this stage of the Pacific War.

Dr. Nagai congratulated me when I reported to him my success in the examination, but he reminded me, "The chest x-ray film at the examination showed a diffuse shadow in the lung. I explained to the testing staff about your last film, which was normal except for a scar, and you were allowed to be a medical student under my supervision."

Before leaving the Nagasaki Regiment, I asked my colleague to delay my second draft until I graduated from the medical school. I did not want to be called again to the army in the middle of my study, as Mr. Fukushima was in Doshisha.

My second eldest brother and his family had moved to Nagasaki from Saga, because he had resigned from his teaching job at a primary school and found work at the Mitsubishi Shipyard. They rented a house near my father's shop and provided a room for me. I moved from my father's house and occupied a room on the second floor of my brother's house. My sister-in-law had been kind to me since my childhood and was happy to have me in her house.

My dream of studying medicine came to reality at last, five years after I read the book by Dr. Albert Schweitzer, who had inspired me. I thanked God for this unexpected privilege.

My days in Nagasaki Medical School started in September, 1943. On the first day, the Dean, Professor Tsunowo, emphasized the seriousness of the present status of the war, and asked us to finish the four-year curriculum of medical study in three or three and a half years, giving up all vacations in spring and summer. Already on the next day the teaching of human anatomy started with dissection of the human corpse assigned to every pair of students. The smell of formalin was unbearable, and dissection of the human body was hard work. There were two professors of anatomy. Professor Yoshito Ikeda was an amiable person, but Professor Jungoro Takaki was a passionate instructor. We were scared by his sharp questions and staring eyes. We had to study Latin to understand anatomical and medical terms derived from Latin.

To my surprise, the teacher of German language was Professor Iwamoto who used to teach us in Saga High School. I did not know what made him leave Saga to become a professor at Nagasaki Medical School. Anyway, I had no escape. I had to attend his class faithfully as his former student. I prepared for each German language class so that I could translate the sentence into Japanese whenever I was asked to do it. It was good for me, because it improved my knowledge of the German language and made my reading of German medical textbooks easier.

Among eighty new medical students there were some who had taken non-science courses in the past. Makoto Mochizuki was one of them. He had graduated from Saga High School in 1943, five years after my graduation, and had studied the liberal arts and German language there. He was a sensitive young son of a family physician in Kagoshima. We found a good friend in each other.

The only old friend among my classmates was Muneo Araki, who had been in the same class in my primary school days, and had been my playmate. We went to the same middle school. We were baptized at the same church and studied at Doshisha, too. He had switched to the medical course, as I had, and we entered Nagasaki Medical School in the same year, a strange coincidence. I did not know, however, that he was destined to die in the middle of his study.

# 42

# THE HILL OF SAINTS

On the first Sunday of 1945, I opened the door of the Furumachi Church, a Presbyterian church, because I wanted to listen to the sermon of Rev. Sonoda of this church.

Since my return from the army, I had attended the Congregational Church where I was baptized in 1932. I had my own Bible class for the adults before the Sunday service. The trouble started when some people attended only my Bible class and did not stay for the Sunday service. Rev. Aoyama was unhappy about it and suggested that I discontinue my Bible class. Others asked me to continue the class. Perplexed, I resigned from the church and started a Bible study meeting on Sunday at my brother's house at the request of my sister-in-law.

I must admit that I was influenced by the writings of Toraji Tsukamoto, a disciple of Kanzo Uchimura who wrote a book entitled in English *How I Became a Christian* and started "Mukyoukai," non-churchism, in Japan. They insist that the invisible ecclesia is not confined to the organized church or sects. According to them, unauthorized lay persons can conduct a Sunday meeting and study and teach the Bible without a church building. The Bible is the only foundation and standard of the ecclesia. The clerical system, sacrament, baptism and all other ceremonies and regulations are unnecessary. A man can be saved only by faith in the Savior who died on the cross for our sins. That was the radical belief of the non-churchists who think they have reached the logical conclusion of Martin Luther's reformation.

Anyway, I was disgusted by the recent change in Japanese churches, where special prayer meetings were held to "win this sacred war against the United States and her allies."

Only three women attended my Sunday morning meeting: my sister-in-law, a widow and a teacher of English. The meeting was simple. It began with hymn singing, followed by my interpretation of the New Testament text, and ended in prayer. It was a warm, sincere meeting. We met every Sunday and studied the gospels and Pauline epistles. My brother did not attend the meeting. He said he had to work on Sunday in this wartime Japan. He might have hesitated to sit and listen to a 15-years younger brother's lesson. But I noticed a subtle change in his attitude toward me. I lived and ate in his house without paying costs, and yet I was using his home as my meeting place, as if it belonged to me, What hurt him most was the attitude of my sister-in-law, who looked at me with respect and affection as her spiritual leader. He criticized our meeting from his Episcopal viewpoint. He had been baptized at an Episcopal church in Nagasaki when he was young. I announced that I would close the meeting at the end of the year, and left his house to go back to my father's newly rented house in Shindaiku Street.

I wanted to listen to a good sermon from a good minister. That was why I visited the Furumachi Church. I was sick of eloquent sermons emphasizing bravery and devotion to the fighting nation. I remembered a simple, plain sermon by Rev. Sonoda which I heard many years ago in a humble, Japanese-style church with the name of "The Church of the Hill of Saints."

Nobody was on the porch. After a few seconds appeared a woman of middle age. She saw me and said, "Please come in." As I entered the chapel, I looked around but could not see anyone inside the chapel.

"Don't you have a service today?" I asked.

"Yes, we do. Please take a seat and wait for a while."

I sat on a front bench as I was told. The ceiling of the chapel was high, and there was stained glass in the window, quite different from what I saw last time.

I had waited for some time, but there came no pastor. The pastor might not be here this morning. He might be working in some other place. The lady looked embarrassed.

"May I conduct the service?" I asked, and stood up in front of the two people. I selected a hymn and we sang together. Then I opened the Bible and read: *"But we know that to them that love God all things work together for good, even to them that are called according to his purpose." (Romans 8:28)*

I confessed that these words contain the wonderful truth which was manifested in my own life. Once a man learned how to love God, then every disadvantage turns to his advantage and leads to happiness in life; lack of money, lack of good family, unexpected hardship and persecution, all turn to good, believe it or not. It is not easy to love God. We can love Him only because He called us, invited us and worked on us. It is Providence. It is Grace. A secret of life for which I cannot be thankful enough. The more I learn, the more grateful I feel.

After my comments we sang a hymn called "Providence" written by Martha A. Cook in 1870 and composed by Philip Phillips.

Thereafter, I went to the Furumachi Church every Sunday. Rev. Sonoda and his family had left Nagasaki in the previous year and there was no pastor in the church. Christianity was regarded as a dangerous"American religion" and people did not dare to approach a church. Many Christians left the church to prove that they were not American spies. A number of pastors were drafted into the army. Many other pastors moved from the city to the safer small towns and villages. Regular Sunday services were not held in most churches in Nagasaki. The Furumachi Church was an exception. My presence on every Sunday was welcomed by the few attending members of the church. The congregation had only five or less attendants!

I found another "Hill of Saints" in Urakami. If one walks from the Nagasaki Medical School toward the northeast, passing by the Urakami Cathedral, he will find a road leading to a Catholic graveyard and then to the "*Jujika-yama*," the Hill of the Cross, which has the Road to Golgotha. In the middle of the slope is located the First Urakami Hospital. Dr. Akizuki described this hill in his book, *A Concentric Death Circle:*

"There is a small hill called the Hill of the Cross on the northeastern edge of Nagasaki. It is nothing but a low hill where wheat and potatoes were planted, but Urakami Catholics regarded this hill as a sacred hill reminding them of the Hill of Golgotha, and prayed here generation after generation throughout the three centuries of persecution from 1587 to 1873.

At the top of the hill stands a big Cross, which was built when Urakami Christians came home from the long exile after freedom of faith was decreed by the new Meiji government. This is a sacred hill revered not only by Catholics in Urakami but also by pilgrims from the Catholic islands to the west of Nagasaki. On the slope below the Cross there stood a French-style building with a red roof. This was the Catholic Theological Seminary. The red bricks of the building reflected the light of the setting sun in the evening, a reminder of the color of the martyr's blood to listeners to the bell of Angelus."

On December 8, 1941, immediately after the attack on Pearl Harbor, all non-Japanese priests and brothers, including Dean Father Prudent, were arrested by the police, and the Theological Seminary was closed. By the efforts of Father Inamochi and Brother Iwanaga, permission to use the building as a sanatorium was granted. The First Urakami Hospital was opened in March, 1942 without a resident doctor. Dr. Takahara visited the sanatorium to see the patients every day, but it was much later in September, 1944, that Dr. Akizuki was stationed in the hospital as a resident physician.

As a medical student who had had a long concern about tuberculosis, I visited the First Urakami Hospital as soon as I learned of this sanatorium early in 1945. Dr. Akizuki was another graduate of Saga High School, two years older than I. He welcomed me and took me around the hospital, introducing me to the chief nurse, Miss Fukahori, and a nurse named Miss Sugako Murai. Miss Fukahori was a Catholic, but Miss Murai was a Protestant who studied at Kassui Mission School and the St. Luke School of Nursing. Dr. Akizuki was a Buddhist, as Dr. Takahara was. It was a staff of interesting combination.

There was a chapel and a room for the Brothers. Brother Iwanaga welcomed me with a big smile. Another Brother named Noguchi was a tuberculosis patient, but he helped with the work of the staff. A Korean Father Paul Ishikawa was the only priest in the hospital. It was a hill of strange saints.

The saint I respected most among them was Dr. Takahara, whose patient I had been. He used to visit the hospital every day from his clinic in Ginyamachi, until Dr. Akizuki came here as a resident doctor. Still, Dr. Takahara made a rounds visit of all patients once a week. On the day of his visit, I came from the medical school to this hospital and visited patients with him and Dr. Akizuki. I listened carefully to their conversation with the patients.

He explained to me the findings on the x-ray films. My interest in tuberculosis increased, making my mind set to become a physician for tuberculosis patients. I was anxious to help them in the near future.

It was Miss Miwa Hirakawa who took care of the empty parsonage after Rev. Sonoda and his family left Nagasaki. She was a younger sister of Mrs. Sonoda. She was the deaconess and treasurer of the poor church, and was responsible for cleaning it all by herself. The wartime duties in the neighborhood were hard work for her. She also took care of invalid boarders in a second floor room, because she could not refuse the request made on behalf of sick people to use the empty parsonage. The newly married wife of Mochizuki, my classmate, was one of those who needed a quiet place to rest.

I was asked by Miss Hirakawa and other deacons of the church to move into the parsonage, because the Army and the local government were looking for vacant houses to commandeer for soldiers and recruited factory workers. I agreed and moved to the parsonage from my father's house. It was good timing for me, because I did not want to be a burden to my father who had to live on the sparse money sent from my brother in Nanjing. I had no payment from the church for my Sunday service, but Miss Hirakawa prepared every meal for me. I did not realize that all expenses were paid by her, not by the church. The meals were as good as the living conditions. I was content. My nieces who came back from Nanjing and were living with my father also enjoyed their visit to the parsonage, staying a week or two in turn. Miss Hirakawa took care of them without complaint.

The South Pacific islands of Saipan, Guam, and Tinian fell to American forces already in 1944. The last resistance of the Japanese soldiers was on the first of March, 1945. The shadow of defeat was heavy over Japan, as the first massive air raid destroyed a large area of Tokyo on the 9th of March. The long dead-heat battle in Okinawa started in April. It was not long before we learned of the death of my sixth elder brother in the Navy. When the news reached my father, he cried aloud in deep sorrow.

The bombing of Kyushu by B29s increased in frequency. Eleven emergency rescue teams of doctors and students were set up in the medical school. Mochizuki and I belonged to the same squad and were stationed in the Department of Ophthalmology, where we gathered as soon as we heard the warning siren, which often sounded after we went home. On many blackout nights I hurried from the parsonage to the medical school hospital on the long dark road. I cannot forget the beauty of the new moon hanging over the complete darkness of the city.

Our running to the hospital was useless every time. The target of the B29s was not our city. It was the Navy factory and the airport in Omura, 20 miles from Nagasaki. We were no longer surprised by the regular visits of the B29s but watched the sky and admired the beautiful big bombers every day, until two bombs were dropped onto the hospital building on the first of August. The building of the departments of Rhinology, Surgery and Gynecology were destroyed by the bombing, and several students were killed.

There was a rumor that local people had picked up leaflets proclaiming that "Nagasaki, a beautiful city of flowers, will be in ashes on the 9th of August." It was a possibility, because on the morning of the 8th, our Dean Professor Tsunowo arrived at the school from Tokyo and told us students what he had seen on his way:

"On the morning of the 6th, we were ordered to leave the train before we reached Hiroshima and we walked along the railroad tracks through the city of Hiroshima. The city was completely destroyed and filled with fire and smoke. A new bomb of enormous power must have been dropped on Hiroshima. We must be prepared for such an eventuality."

Everyone caught their breath as he finished his report.

On the next day, at 11:02 a.m., a plutonium bomb was dropped on the city of Nagasaki from a height of 8,000 meters above the ground.

# 43

# THE CLOUD AND THE LIGHT

I love the scene of a dramatic sky, when a stream of light comes through the cloud and falls on the sea, connecting the sky and the sea with a string of light. The shining ripples of waves enlighten the whole dark ocean. I saw such a scene on the Shimabara Peninsula on the way from Unzen west to Obama, which overlooks the ocean. I saw it to the north in Ariake Bay and also in Omura Bay, north beyond Nagasaki. But the most impressive view of the drama of the cloud and the light was the one I saw over Tachibana Bay on a scenic seaside road running from the Shimabara Peninsula toward Nagasaki. Suddenly from the dark evening sky a string of light ran out of the cloud toward the water like an arrow of light. Immediately a ring of waves reflected the light and sent it back to the sky like sparkling stars. It reminds me of a phrase in the Bible, *"It will become brighter in the evening."* And it reminded me of the picture of Jesus praying in Gesthemane which I saw in the Riverside Church near the Hudson River. He was sitting in prayer with his eyes looking at the light coming through the thick cloud. Such a drama of the cloud and the light always reminds me of the moment when I found a dim light in the middle of the cloud of the atomic bomb. I walked toward the light and found the window from which I jumped out to a new destiny in life.

There are times of darkness in life. There are many scenes of darkness. We look for the light. We wait for the light. We put our hope on the light coming through the cloud. We entrust our life to a stream of light penetrating the cloud. I was one of those who hope. When I felt lonely in my childhood without enough care and enough money, I found a quiet joy in reading books. In the world of fairy tales and fictions I forgot the reality of sorrow and loneliness and built up my own dream. I found a new light coming from heaven in the church which I happened to enter. It was a revelation from a different world. I have read the Bible to find the secret message in it. This strange document written in a foreign land was not easy to understand, but there were words in it filled with instruction and inspiration. At first they sounded strange and impracticable. But they became a good guide for life and gave light to the darkness of life, if one followed obediently and practised faithfully. The life guided by the light may look foolish and unhappy sometimes, but it is bound to the sky with an invisible string of blessing. And an indescribable happiness flows into the life.

I had never expected to get a higher education, but I was allowed to study at a middle school, a privilege denied to my six brothers. I did not expect to pass the entrance examination to high school, but I had the luck to study at Saga High School. When I could not get any more support from my father to continue my study, kind help was offered to me. I experienced illness and surgery, but I learned lessons from the experience. My dream of studying theology in Doshisha University was interrupted by my illness and disillusionment, and I had to labor in Manchuria for three years as a soldier. If I had stayed in Doshisha, I would have been drafted at the last stage of the war and sent to a miserable battlefield in Burma or the Philippines to be killed in battle. I respected Dr. Albert Schweitzer, but I never expected to have an opportunity to become a doctor myself. After finishing service in the army I was accepted as a medical student in the Nagasaki Medical School, because I met a doctor in the army who taught me how to succeed in the entrance examination. It was by Providence, and the same Providence worked on the ninth of August and saved me miraculously from the tragedy of the atomic bomb.

I often asked myself "What should I do as a man who was saved from the fate of death?" and I found answers whenever I needed them. I should say that the answers were given to me. My first duty as a doctor was to save people from tuberculosis of the lung, because it was the major killer of the Japanese in the war-stricken, defeated nation. To accomplish my work, I had to study pulmonary surgery in the United States. When tuberculosis lost its menace and head injuries increased in the automobile age, my second duty was to start neurosurgery in our University Hospital. It was also by Providence that I found a neurosurgical residency at the University of Oregon Medical School.

When the Department of Neurosurgery was approved by the government a dozen years later in Nagasaki, I was not appointed head of the Department, but another duty was waiting for me in Kita-kyushu. Reconstruction of Yahata City Hospital, setting up of the medical emergency center, and the "Kita-kyushu Life Line"— they all needed me. The unexpected diagnosis of lung cancer and the death of my brother drove me to a new, difficult war against smoking. I put all my energy and enthusiasm into each task. All my efforts were not in vain. I left Kita-kyushu with satisfaction. The Yahata Hospital changed to a fine, large hospital. The old deficit had changed to a new surplus. The waiting room is crowded with many outpatients now, five times what it was when I started. The telephone of the "Kita-kyushu Life Line" rings day and night and changes despair into hope. The fire of the anti-smoking movement spread all over Japan, and the 6th World Conference on Smoking and Health and the International Symposium for a Smoke-free New Century were invited to Japan. In my retired life in Nagasaki I am still bound to many people with warm friendship. I feel I am blessed. All these blessings are the result of my single-minded struggle to accomplish what I regarded as an order from God. I have just followed the destiny assigned by my Heavenly Father.

But I feel sorry for Miwa who volunteered to be my lifetime partner. Her life was an endless hardship, because I devoted myself to my work and cared little about the income to support her. She supported me by her sewing. She spent little for herself and saved money to buy the books I needed. She stayed at home and patiently waited for my return during my study abroad, five years in total, exactly as St. Paul described the Christian life when he wrote, *"Love is patient."* He also wrote, *"Love is kind; love is not jealous or boastful; it is not arrrogant or rude. Love does not insist on its own way; it is not irritable or resentful; it does not rejoice at wrong, but rejoices in the right. Love bears all things, believes all things, hopes all things, endures all things."* All these descriptions fit Miwa. I agree when anyone tells me, "Everything that you are now you owe to the help of your wife."

Miwa is ninety years old now in 1996, fifty years after our marriage. She cannot walk well since she broke her right leg four years ago. Now she is in bed because she broke her ankle this summer. She cannot be well forever. I have to watch her becoming weaker, ill, and sick. The time of permanent separation is inevitable. It is a painful thought. Neither am I proof against death.

Everyone fears death. Nothing is more sad than separation from one's dear ones. It is a universal human nature to fear death and seek for eternal life. Nevertheless, our physical body will come to the end of its activity.

We fear death because we are afraid of the agony before death and because we are afraid of an unknown future after death. We are grateful to medicine, because pain as well as anxiety can be relieved by proper medication. When I visited St. Joseph Hospice in London, nobody looked sad or in pain. Everyone was enjoying life, even though many of the patients knew that their life in this world was almost over. I could not forget their happy faces when they chatted with their visiting family or friends. Though their happy state was mainly the effect of a medication called the Brompton cocktail, it also resulted from the good care and smiles of the nurses, doctors and volunteers who worked there. When the last moment approaches, there is no tracheotomy, artificial respiration, cardiac massage, injection after injection in this hospice. Instead, a family or friend, or doctor, or nurse, sits next to the dying one, holding his or her hand and watching the eyes. The patient slowly opens the eyes, looks at the dear one close to him, and again closes the eyes with satisfaction and trust. It is a scene of peace and of happiness.

According to Raymond Moody, the author of *Life after Death* (1975), the common experience of 150 persons who nearly died was "a feeling of passing through a long dark tunnel at enormous speed," "and, suddenly {slipping} out of the physical body," "then, the presence of souls of dead relatives and friends nearby.... Finally the presence of a glorious life filled with love and warmth, a life of brilliant light."

It reminded me of the experience I had on an airplane. The earth was dark and in rain. But after flying up and up through the thick clouds, suddenly opened a wide, bright blue sky. All the clouds were now below the plane, brilliantly reflecting the sunshine like an Alpine range of snow-white mountains. It was a miraculous transformation of the dark clouds to sunny brilliance. It was a breath-taking view of an astonishing beauty, out of this world. The sky kept its brightness until late in the evening in the northern flight. Light pink and golden colors filled the sky and a feeling of previously unexperienced happiness filled my heart. I might have had a glimpse of the world after death.

Watching the sky of deep blue
Peace and rest fill my soul.

A massive cloud of sunny white
Flows from the east to the west
Chased by the cloud of grey

Followed by the other clouds
Changing the color of the clouds
Passing through the wide heaven.

After the clouds comes the sky
With another deeper blue
Staining my soul in deeper blue.

Then the pink and golden color
Illuminates the whole sky
Before the scarlet curtain falls.

And the peace of unknown blue
Spreads to my soul in heaven.